SKIN DEEP

SKIN DEEP

ROBERT HELMER, M.D.

NASH PUBLISHING
LOS ANGELES

Library of Congress Catalog Card Number: 76-167512
Standard Book Number: 8402-1207-0

Published simultaneously in the United States and Canada
by Nash Publishing Corporation, 9255 Sunset Boulevard,
Los Angeles, California 90069.

Printed in the United States of America

First Printing

This book is respectfully dedicated to my father, Richard W. Helmer, a compassionate, gentlemanly scholar who imbued my brothers and me with a spirit and a desire to understand and communicate with our fellow man, regardless of station or circumstance, and a tolerance for the ideas, manners, and dispositions of others.

My thanks to my editor, Brett Howard, and to the many dermatological sources of invaluable research which we had at our disposal for composing *Skin Deep*.

CONTENTS

THE BAG YOU LIVE IN

This book is a treatise for you and your skin.

Skin: that incredible, miraculous, integumentary investiture, the elastic covering in which the Creator of all things encased the image of Himself.

Skin is the largest organ of the human body, holding within its flexible form all of the other organs which constitute a living being. Not only is it a container of important and sometimes essential parts which make the image more functional and more readily manifest, but it is also a reflective mirror of the elusive, sensitive, incorporeal essence of the mind, the soul. It is a station of communication whereby the internal organs can be signalled of the necessity of making adjustments to changing environment.

Skin, for the maintenance of its outward appearance, nets more than one billion, five million dollars annually to the cosmetic industry, in the United States alone.

There are more than 2,100 separate skin diseases and there are today more than 3,000 licensed doctors of medicine specializing in the study of skin care.

You can live without your arms, your legs, your sight, your hearing, and in this day of transplants, you can survive, with the surgical installation of many artificial, substitute organs. But, if a large portion of your skin is destroyed, you will die. It therefore seems important that each individual should know as much as possible about one of the most important organs of the human body, an organ which for centuries has been taken for granted.

The versatile, ever-changing skin commences to take form in the early months of fetal development, being closely related from the start to your central nervous system. When you emerge from your mother's womb, you are wrapped in the skin with which you will have to live and in which you will one day die. It will assume different forms and appearances throughout your lifetime, but even in death it will retain its solid cellular form. At birth, your mother touches the bag containing the solid, living creature which has been created within her body and she welcomes the newborn child into the world with love, which becomes the first mode of communication. Speech comes two or three years later, as it did proportionately two or three eons later in the evolutionary process of man. But before speech there exists the communication of the loving, protective, soft embrace of the parent—or, the coarse, cruel, noncaressing touch of rejection. From the moment of birth until the hour of death your skin is a tell-tale symbol of your reactions to the acceptance of life and living, or your eventual adjustment to the first spurning of the same external forces employed in negation. You might blush with embarrassment, become livid in anger or pallid in fear.

Despite the physiological and psychological importance of skin, most people are only concerned with the superficial value of the largest and one of the most important organs with which they live.

In the beginning, after the creation of Heaven and Earth, Adam encountered Eve and liked what he saw. He touched the bag in which she lived; she touched the forbidden fruit and enticed him to eat of it; and both were expelled from the Garden of Eden. In their shame, they partially clothed their naked bodies, a gesture which has evolved into an enduring custom. After the deluge, only Noah and his three sons—Shem, Ham, and Japheth—remained. Ham beheld the nakedness of his father and was accursed for his indiscretion. Shem was the supposed progenitor of the Hebrews, the Arabs, Assyrians, Babylonians, Phoenicians, and so forth; Japheth of the European and near-Asiatics. It was Cush, however, one of the sons of Ham, who offers the first definite instance of the mention of race. Cush is the Hebrew word for black, and Ethiopia was the habitat of his descendants.

From these forebears, the Biblical peoples migrated across the world and encountered, much to their amazement, other faces, other places. Somehow there emerged (historically with the Cynics of Athens) the philosophy which has been vaguely expressed as "all men being created equal," and "brothers under the skin."

Scientifically, however, the variations of skin pigmentations between you and your brother, as well as your other traits and characteristics, are established genetically, under the aegis of the Supreme Being. How and where the different races originated with color alterations is still quite moot.

For the purpose of orientation in learning about your skin, I will define a few terms and structures.

Your skin is basically divided into the *epidermis,* or scarf skin, and the *dermis,* or corium, called the true skin. The *epidermis* is without blood vessels or nerves, is constantly dying and being reborn, in a process which begins in the inner layers and grows outward. The following layers are recognized in the *epidermis:* an outermost layer of horny material of variable thickness called the *stratum corneum.* The deepest portion of this layer is referred to as the "barrier area," termed the *stratum lucidum* in the palms and soles, where it is particularly prominent. The "barrier area" is so called because of its remarkable role as a protective shield for all the functioning elements of your body. It is a super sheath and its effectiveness has been clearly illustrated in its affinity to rebuff such noxious elements as the poisonous gases used in World War I and the present-day pollutants of the atmosphere. All of these can be readily injurious when introduced through the relatively small portals of the eyes, nose, and mouth, but they encounter an almost impenetrable electrochemical wall of resistance to passage through your skin "barrier." The cellular layer beneath the stratum corneum is prominent because it contains unique blue-staining granules and is called the *stratum granulosum.* Below this granular layer lies the *stratum mucosum*—generally the thickest portion of the epidermis—a mosaic of actively multiplying cells firmly bound one to another. Its base consists of a single layer of palisaded cells called the *stratum germinativum,* the

CROSS SECTION OF SKIN

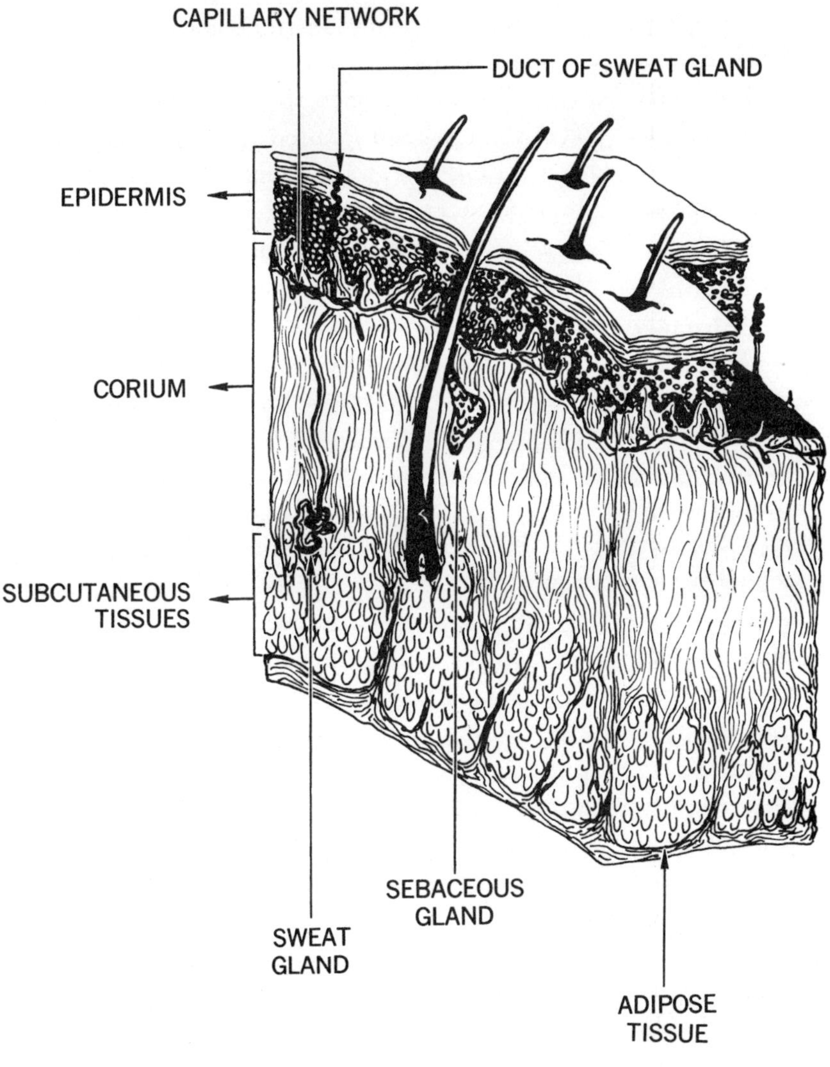

innermost layer of the epidermis, from which the other layers of the epidermis ultimately derive, moving in progression toward the surface while changing their characteristics in the several layers, eventually being sloughed off as dry dander. This is known as the *cornification* process. It is self renewing, flexible, and constantly changing. When the cells of the mother layer—the *stratum germinativum*—are destroyed, they are irreplaceable, and scarring results. The area where the epidermal cells meet the more loosely constructed dermis is known as the *dermal-epidermal junction.* In the dermis there are multitudes of fingerlike projections which protrude into the substance of the overlying epidermis, and by means of which the two primary components of the skin are dowelled together, held in tenacious proximity by a remarkable cement, the strength of which has never been approximated in the laboratories of man.

The *dermis,* the source of strength and elasticity of the skin, contains connective tissue fibers, cellular elements and ground substance, and is the repository of the countless nerve endings and organs of sensation for the perception of touch, of pain, of warmth and cold; and also of the sweat glands, the oil glands, hair follicles, and other strategic "epidermal appendages."

In addition, the epidermis is covered with a lubricating film of the residual products of cornification and of the excretions of those superficial glands just mentioned, a "magic mantle," which is of itself highly protective.

In reading about skin you will discover that in the language of the poet the adjectives silky, velvety, dewy prevail and skin is ivory or waxen, or it might glow with the rosy fingers of dawn, or bronze with the golden hue of sunset; but it usually has to be *white* to be termed *beautiful.* The phrases of these enthusiastic poets and lovers inspire efforts to fulfill their ideals. Ladies have been known to cover their faces with heavy applications of white chalk *maquillage,* such as the masters of clown make-up apply to create their comic effects.

Incredibly, this outlandish cosmetic procedure was employed not only by fair-skinned Caucasian ladies, but by black-skinned Ethiopian beauties, Japanese Geisha girls and Shinto brides, and certain ruddy American Indian heroines.

Eventually, color was added to the basic white. Classical Greek beauties, influenced no doubt by Sappho of Lesbos, were the progenitors of exposure to the sun's rays, walking, as they did, sandal-footed and bare-armed through the streets of Athens while the bright Aegean sun filtered through their flowing garments and highlighted their high-boned cheeks.

Later, the ladies of the Renaissance, inspired by new techniques for the portrayal of light, perspective and color, applied some of the paint tones from the artist's palette and the colors of their skins went from Florentine rose to Venetian chrome yellow. But, for the most part, the lavish praise of the verbal connoisseurs of skin beauty sang aloud the Arthurian glories of "Elaine the fair, Elaine, the lily maid of Astolat," as in Tennyson's "Idylls of the King." Consequently, the epitome of skin beauty was the traditional fair-skinned English lass whose peaches-and-cream complexion was the envy of the women of the world. The Gainsborough beauties were endemic of a skin culture of porcelain fragility, heralded by the painted porcelain face of Elizabeth, the Virgin Queen.

It has only been in recent years that other skin colors have procured honorable mention among the beauty worshippers, although many famous women in history—notably Cleopatra, Queen of Egypt, and Josephine, wife of Napoleon Bonaparte, Empress of France and grandmother of Napoleon III—have possessed dark complexions.

With the growing respect commanded by the African nations, black people the world over have begun to appreciate their native beauty and to glorify it. At this writing, the African look is very "in," not only in fashion, but in skin coloring, make-up, and "natural" hair styles. Black-cosmetic firms have mushroomed into successful business enterprises, manufacturing appropriate color cosmetics for skins ranging in color from sepia to ebony. The result is certainly more esthetic than the previous grotesque application of white skin powders and outrageous lip colors to dark-complexioned persons. The beauty of such actresses as Lena Horne, Diahann Carroll and Leslie Uggams and the virility and handsome mien of actors like Harry Belafonte and Sidney Poitier has had an appreciable effect upon the purveyors of skin pulchritude.

Since World War II, Caucasian men and women have circulated so that there is a markedly different attitude now toward the various skin pigmentations of the sundry races. We have commingled and cohabited to create a new look, possibly a new color—a sort of international *cafe au lait.* But, because the color of your skin is determined by multiple genes with cumulative effect, there is not now nor is there likely to be an overall universal color of the human race.

The dominant light wave length of your skin color is in the region of 589 milli-microns, or sodium yellow. Individual color depends upon the thickness and transparency of the upper epidermal layers, blood content and distribution of blood vessels, amount and arrangement of the subcutaneous fat, and amount and distribution of pigments which include melanoid, carbon, reduced hemoglobin, oxyhemoglobin, and principally *melanin.*

Melanin is believed by some to be a heritage of our prehuman, anthropoid ancestry. Its formation begins with the oxidation of the amino acid *tyrosine* under the catalytic action of the copper-containing enzyme *tyrosinase.*

In both the human and the animal world we find the *albino* skin which is equipped with a normal number of *melanocytes,* or pigment cells, but it suffers from a defect in the enzymatic activity which prevents the pigment formation, so that, as a consequence, color is absent.

Tyrosinase in its normal state is partially inhibited. Sunlight, X-rays, and alpha particles remove the inhibitors, thereby permitting increased pigment formation. The pigment then absorbs much of the radiation which would otherwise harm sensitive skin cells.

It is not merely the greater number of melanocytes in dark-skinned people which produces the color difference, but the higher proportion of melanin and its distribution in the upper dermal layers and in the *stratum germativum.* One theory describes color change in mankind as both evolutionary and geographical. It presumes that when the descendants of the Neanderthal man began to lose body hair in order to adapt themselves to tropical climates, the melanin that formerly colored the hair concentrated into the skin and incidentally served as a beneficial adaptation to strong sunlight. Fanciful but of interest.

Exposure of the entire body to the sun to acquire the radiant, supposedly healthy look of sun tan is comparatively recent. Originally, only the face, hands and arms and very little of the chest were ever exposed to the sun. The result was limited tanned areas. One lady patient of mine once confessed that she had never beheld anything so white as the torso of a rugged, sun tanned cowboy whose only exposure to the sun involved his head and face, arms and forearms. It left a vivid impression on this jet-setter who had languished in the sun from the shores of St. Tropez to the beach at Waikiki in a bare bikini and had never before encountered such a figure, bronzed of face and limb, but whose nude, previously unexposed parts were pure white.

Actually, the sunning of the entire body is closely related to *the* fashionable disease of the nineteenth century—the dread tuberculosis. At that time, the treatment was rest in a high altitude and exposure to the sun's rays. A European patient returning to foggy London town after his recuperative stay at Thomas Mann's *Magic Mountain* presents an exuberant picture of health. The wan, dying consumptive ladies and gentlemen of pallor began to retire. Their whiteness indicated a smouldering, decadent disease within or an economic inability to enjoy a season in the sun. Sun coloring became an economic and class identity-symbol. The very social and the very rich enjoyed the color of the sun reflected on their bodies, while the poor, lower-class individual was grey and drab, chained to his office routine in the smoky, grimy cities of the industrial age. Unfortunately, the sun worshippers were not properly indoctrinated in the sun's miseries as well as the sun's joys, and in time many paid an exorbitant price of irreparable skin damage for the change in the pigmentation of the skin.

In both embryology and evolution, skin is the body's

oldest sensory and reactive structure. It shares a common origin with the nervous system; consequently, diseases of your skin are closely allied to your nervous system. Both develop from the *ectoderm* (the outermost layer of the developing embryo). The central nervous system and the organs of special senses all commence as special infoldings of the embryonic "skin."

The bag you live in, being the protector of your inner organs, is essentially a tough, elastic bag which is self-repairing, self-cleansing, and provides its own germicidal excretions.

Your skin comprises about 6 percent of your body weight, averaging about ten pounds for men and seven for women. In thickness, it is about three to four millimeters—two-tenths of an inch—on the back and about 0.3 millimeters—one one-hundreth of an inch—on the eyelids. Approximately one third of your bloodstream flows through your skin.

Your skin has about two million sweat glands which share with your lungs about a quart of water per day for cooling by evaporation. In short, you are your own "built-in air conditioner." In a day the average adult skin area of between nineteen and twenty-one square feet dissipates around two thousand, five hundred calories—enough to boil twenty quarts of water. Loose texture, large sweat glands, plentiful sebaceous oily secretions and sparse body hair are among the skin's cooling devices. The vascular thermostatic control is apparently by means of the arteriolar system. Hot- or cold-sensitive nerve endings initiate the thermostatic reflex mechanisms in response to environmental temperature changes. Normally these are integrated through the hypothalamus, involuntarily, unless other activities such as muscular action or sexual participation require a more complex regulatory system involving the more involved mechanisms of the central nervous system. In short, when we work out in a gym or in a bedroom, our body temperature requires special conditioning, much in the same manner as we adjust our mechanical air-conditioning units—up or down—by thermostatic control to fit the room's temperature to the congeniality of its inhabitants.

Until very recently, comfort and beauty were the two chief concerns humans had regarding the bag in which they lived. One approached the subject of the enormous organ which would house the inner person throughout life almost like an advertising agency executive packaging a new product for the market.

One commiserated with people who had bad skin, but little was done to 1) understand why the skin was "bad" or, 2) what to do medically or individually to remedy the ill. As our understanding and compassion has developed, we tend to study the life of a man such as Jean Paul Marat, one of the leaders of the French Revolution, and we observe that his personal life and perhaps the course of history might have been altered had anyone known about, or been able to offer a remedy for, his wretched skin condition. The agony of the tortures of his skin is attested to in the occurrence of his assassination at the hands of Charlotte Corday, who killed him while he sat in a tub of warm oil trying to relieve the miserable itching of his body covered with eczema.

Today we are finally alerted to the close physiological and emotional affinity between the skin and the inner being. We are conscious that this miraculous "bag" is our protective covering, adjusting as the animal's furry coat adjusts to environmental hazards. We are beginning to penetrate, medically and philosophically, the nature of skin and its most important role in man's relation to himself and to his fellow man.

Your skin is your best—or worst—salesman. It speaks for you as volubly as does the organ of speech. It is your first impression; it pleases or repels and it often indicates to the trained observer the possible malfunction of other, nonvisible, organs of your body.

It might be of interest for you to know that the very intensified study of the skin in the field of medicine—the specialty of dermatology—is itself relatively new. And the progression of the dermatologist to correlating the diseases of the skin to the psyche of his patient is extremely contemporary. Although Hippocrates and the ancients wrote of and described various skin diseases, and the Arabs preserved and elaborated upon their observations for later transmission to the Romans, it was the scourge of leprosy and its manifestations that spread interest in diseases of the skin, and, together with bubonic plague (named for the *buboes* or sores that appear on the skin), occupied a preeminent position in cutaneous medicine until the European arrival of the great mimic of other diseases.

Syphilis spread like wildfire across the continent, beginning in the early sixteenth century and lasting to the present day. From the beginning, the study of the skin and social diseases was closely correlated, primarily because the lesions of the latter are chiefly exhibited in the skin. By the beginning of the nineteenth century, Robert Willan of England had written the first formal classification of diseases of the skin, and shortly thereafter, prominent dermatologists were conducting skin clinics—Baron Jean Louis Alibert at the Hospital

St. Louis in Paris, Ferdinand von Hebra of the Viennese School and our own Henry Daggett Bulkley at the Broome Street Clinic in New York. However, as recently as when I started specializing in the study of the skin (twenty-one years ago), the subject was viewed with much skepticism by those of my colleagues who looked upon themselves as potential brain surgeons or learned professors specializing in the mysteries of the inner organs. Dermatologists were, and to some extent still are, regarded as "frivolous" physicians, because the skin does not necessarily present the emergency of immediate death, and the doctor can adjust his life to some sort of reasonable schedule, not being perpetually "on call." But the attitude of the physicians and of the patient is rapidly changing. You are becoming aware of the importance of your skin in health and disease, in youth and old age, and beyond its appearance and the requirements for bodily comfort. You are beginning to understand the importance of your environment to the health of your skin, and in this day of excess tension you are also becoming cognizant of the effects of emotional stress on your nervous system and the resultant projection onto your skin of the many psychosomatically related dermatoses we see every day.

Our skin has brought mankind with remarkable protective custody to our modern age. But, our skin has never before been in conflict with so many disturbing influences, both from within and without. Our skin has survived plague and pestilence—the great pox (syphilis), the smallpox, the black plague (bubonic) and the white (tuberculosis). It has survived disasters of warfare and combats of sex, but today our skin is vulnerable to an inner enemy, a tension created of and by ourselves, which day after day tends to make itself more

ETIOLOGY OF SKIN DISEASES

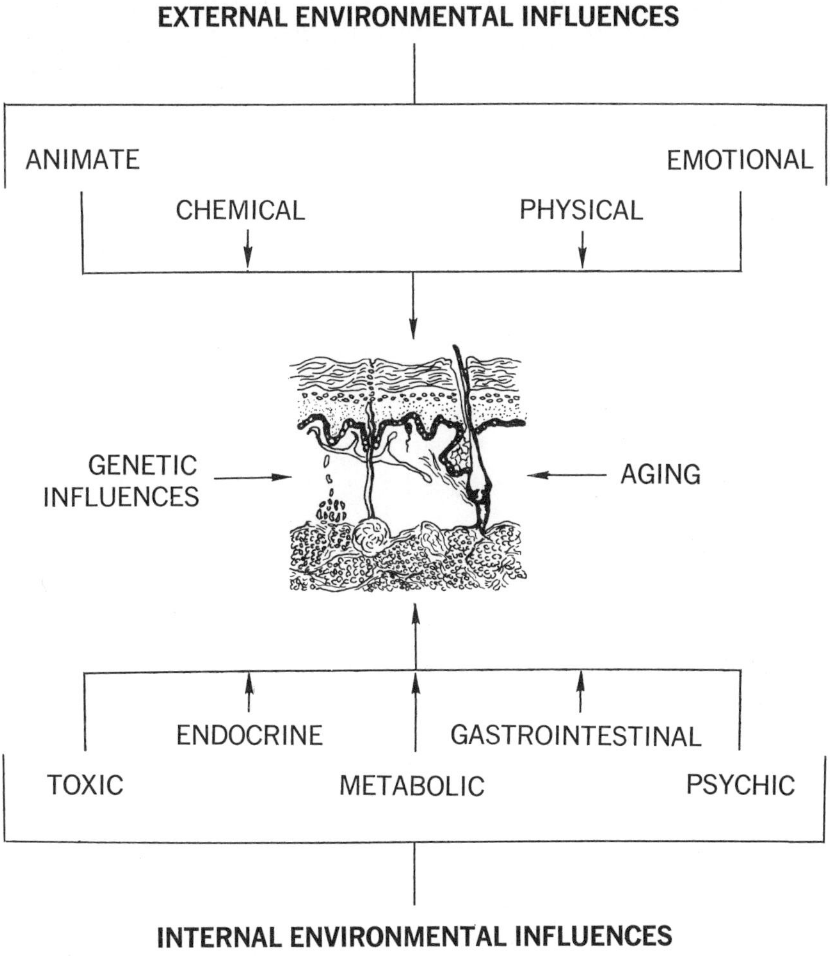

manifest. It is for a wider understanding of the bag you live in—you and your skin—that this book was written. It is an attempt to tell you what a dermatologist knows about your skin upon confrontation and consultation. The resultant is your responsibility, basically. This is your bag, man, as the teenager would say—you've got to live with it as well as within it.

SKIN: THE SENSE ORGAN

"The skin is the barrier as well as the principal organ of communication between the animal and its environment. It is a mirror which reflects the well-being or the disorders of the rest of the organism . . ."

—William Montagna

Once considered with no greater significance than merely "the bag you live in," skin has finally come into its own as a major organ, a gallimaufry of dissimilar tissues performing vital and often mysterious functions for both body and mind. Today, your doctor is concerned with your skin and its relationship with nervous and endocrine systems, the pathways of its interreactions with the psyche that makes it a mirror for the physician to study.

Modern electronic testing equipment reveals that your skin is a sense organ in more senses than previously suspected. Experiments have shown that vibratory impulses transmitted in sentence form by an alphabetic code at the rate of thirty-five-letter words per minute can be received by the skin with 90 percent accuracy. In one test experiment, subjects manipulated a steering wheel in response to cutaneous signals as efficiently as a group controlled by lights.

Vibrators are used on the ventral thorax (chest); codes using different loci, intensities, frequencies, and electric signals within the narrow limits of comfort and safety are also possible on other parts of the body. Experiments with cutaneous communications systems were originally for use with the deaf-blind, but the work of scientists today anticipates situations in which visual and aural reception may be inadequate or impractical. In short, if in our evolutionary process and in our absorption of the earth's living facilities we make the ultimate flight into space and reorient our living in space, skin assumes an even greater importance. Because of its remarkable flexibility, it can possibly protect us as it has since the beginning of time and make the essential adjustments to a new environment.

Your skin is a jungle of eponyms: Pacinian corpuscles for detecting pressure, Meissner's for touch, Krause's end-organs for cold, Ruffini's for appreciating warmth. Only pain enjoys no specialized structure. Its nerve endings accompany each specialized end organ so that intense stimulation of any of the senses produces pain. If your sundry receptors were evenly distributed, each square inch of the body's surface would have twenty-four heat receptors; four for cold, fifty for touch and four hundred pain nerves. Distribution of nerve receptors is highly selective. Cold nerves are most plentiful on your back, heat nerves on the ventral surface.

The palm sides of fingertips have touch nerves so closely

placed that two strokes only fractionally separated can be individually distinguished, but if two objects are felt on the skin of your forearm an inch apart the sensation is one of a single taction.

In the words of the poet, the sense of touch is compared to that of the spider, "The spider's touch, how exquisitely fine! Feels at each thread, and lives along the line." (Pope's *Essay on Man*). Man's touch is referred to in many of the modes of life he selects. The pianist has the touch *pianissimo;* the artist the *touch of genius;* the skilled surgeon, the physician's *healing touch.* Your manual dexterity is controlled by the sense of touch in your fingertips and that original sensitivity is with you at birth. The drummer taps the tight surface of the drum and creates music; the cook touches the dough in the bread and by the texture knows when to bake; the sculptor creates his work of art by sensing the composition of the material in his hand; the lover touches the skin of his beloved and is filled with desire.

In the important area of communication, the sensory nerve of the skin on our fingertips is almost as important as our spoken word. It creates a physical contact upon shaking of the hand of a stranger. The reaction can be good or bad, it connotes much of the inner impression. If the fingertip is wet, or dry, hard or soft, we are alerted to reactions by the contact of the sensory nerves of touch.

Concentrations of nerves surround the base of each hair follicle over the entire skin and the afferent nerve fibers form a continuous network from superficial to deep levels. They transmit a light moving stimulus as a *tickle,* a stronger moving stimulus as *itching,* a still more potent stimulus as *pain.* There are two types of stimulation mediated by two different types of nerves, "fast" pain (so called because of the immediacy of the reaction to the stimulus), carried by insulated nerve fibers, and "slow" pain, carried by noninsulated ones. Fast pain is a sharp, pricking, well-localized pain of short duration. This is followed by a sensationless period, after which begins the slow pain, consisting of a more diffuse, aching or burning sensation. Pricking the skin with a sharp instrument such as a pin will adequately demonstrate these qualities.

The skin's first line of defense against its environment is a thin film of emulsified material spread rather evenly over its entire surface. The components of this complex film are contributed by sebaceous glands, sweat glands, and the products of cornification. Among the contents of this surface film are: lactic acid, amino acids, urea, uric acid, and ammonia derived from sweat glands; triglycerides, free fatty acids and wax alcohols derived from the sebaceous glands; and sterols, amino acids, pentoses, phospholipids, and complex polypeptides derived from the cornification process.

The composition of this film will differ in many different areas of the body and these differences will in many cases determine specific susceptibility of an area to a particular bacterium, fungus or other parasites, as well as determine regional localization of many common skin diseases.

For example, the soles of your feet do not contain sebaceous glands and therefore do not contribute such products as triglycerides, fatty acids and wax alcohols to the surface films of your feet. This fact we doctors correlate to the following facts: 1) that fungus or other parasitic saprophytic blight, as well as other infections, occur commonly on the soles of the feet (almost everyone has encountered athlete's foot at one time or another) but rarely attack the lower part of the leg or the calf area; and 2) unsaturated fatty acids derived from the sebaceous glands are strongly antagonistic to fungi.

A simple example of a disease created by change in the surface film is that seen in the winter dryness of old people's skin. This condition is technically known as *asteatosis* or *xeroderma.*

> "What youth deemed crystal, Age finds out was dew.
> Morn set a-sparkle, but which noon quick dried."
> —Robert Browning "Jochanan Hakkadosh"

What has happened to the "crystal" that age discovers to be "dew?" In technical terms, the supply of lipid substances to the skin surface is insufficient, so the horny layer does not bind water properly, becomes dehydrated, scaly and fissured, with resultant extreme *pruritus* or itching. Contrary to popular belief, it is a lack of water in the skin rather than a deficiency of oil which causes dryness. The natural oils of the skin emulsify and help to bind the water, allowing for a more supple, pliant organ. Excessive extraction of the oils that bind by the prolonged use of solvents or detergents will, therefore, cause a diminution of water in the skin and a drying condition.

The horny layer is a definite, if not complete, physical barrier to electromagnetic waves, microorganisms, parasites, noxious chemicals, and practically all environmental agents. Its principal ingredient is *keratin,* a tough fibrous protein which depends to a great extent on disulfide linkages and hydrogen bonds for its unique resistant properties. It is highly resistant to acid and alkali, as well as common enzymatic proteolytic agents. Where the horny layer meets the granular layer there is a specialized area of keratin which functions as a selective barrier to absorption. Once the barrier area is damaged or removed, practically any molecule regardless of size or other characteristics will easily pass through the cellular epidermis.

The cellular epidermis is the functional protective organ and is the area of skin which blisters upon injury. The blisters may occur at the junction between the dermis and the epidermis, between the germinal layer and the *stratum mucosum,* or in the mucosal layer itself. Actually, over thirty skin diseases, including the quite commonplace poison ivy, involve the formation of skin blisters, the location of the blisters in the layers of the skin depending in many cases on the disease.

Your skin not only protects you but because it encloses you it affords the covering which makes it possible for you to survive in an excessively warm or cold climate. It enables you to change your peripheral blood flow in order to lose or retain body warmth, the former primarily by means of convection. The latter after maximum blood flow has been attained, the body loses heat by means of evaporation, through the sweat mechanism. In a cold environment, after the peripheral blood vessels are constricted to their greatest degree, body temperature is maintained by muscular contractions, or "chills." The subject of sweating is one which was once "verboten" in polite company. Ladies and gentlemen *perspired,* the common folk *sweated.* As Prime Minister Sir Winston Churchill elevated *sweat* to the language of the upper classes when he made his famous statement in the House of Commons in 1940: "I have nothing to offer but blood, toil, tears and sweat." To a world terrified by the onslaught of Nazi Germany conquering continental Europe, the offer of sweat meant hours of heroic slavery. The word sweat invoked honest labor exemplified by sweat upon the brow and the image of fat as illustrated by Shakespeare's Falstaff in *Henry IV,* who "sweats to death and lards the lean earth as he walks along."

Through your sweat mechanism you deliver up to fourteen quarts of sweat per day. This sweat is released through the skin and the organ of sweating consists of three parts: 1) the glandular part deep in the dermis which is responsible for secreting sweat; 2) the dermal portion of the duct which transports sweat; 3) the epidermal portion of the duct which delivers the sweat to the surface of the skin. The importance of sweat to the appearance and care of your skin is analysed later in connection with the odors and diseases connected with the sweat glands. Under no set of circumstances should you ever be embarrassed by your sweat, nor fail to recognize its very vital importance in the life of your skin and your health in general.

It is interesting to note that, although man is a "warm-blooded" creature with a constant body temperature, his nonvascular epidermis is a "cold-blooded" organ, the temperature of which changes with the temperature of the environment. Aside from clothing habits, it is through the intercession of his dermis that man provides an adjustment to the outside temperature and frees himself from the whims and vagaries of weather on which the very existence of reptilian creatures is totally dependent.

In understanding your skin you must recognize that the sun is the skin's *number one* ecologic foe. To convey this truth is the hardest single duty of the dermatologist. To get the patient to accede is equally difficult. And, to believe for one minute that the individual who has never suffered any more damage from the sun's ray than a superficial sunburn will never accept the idea of sun danger is almost preposterous for the doctor to presume or for the layman to concede. Facts are facts and the truth of constant exposure to the sun is evidenced in the coarsening, drying, laxity and wrinkling which are its main degenerative effects. Some protection is available in the use of those cosmetic products which filter out the damaging light wave lengths; products which contain such things as tannic acid, para-aminobenzoic acid, the salicylates, quinine and other chemical parasols. Many persons with reddish or auburn skin or hair coloring are particularly susceptible to the deleterious effects of the sun. Whether or not this is due to the presence of the unique iron-containing reddish-brown pigment found solely in those persons has not been fully established, but, in any case, they should assiduously avoid the sun.

The contrast of the average skin with daily exposure to the sun with one who has assiduously avoided such danger is seldom seen. Recently in my practice I saw a ninety-two-year-old woman who had avoided any exposure to the sun during her entire lifetime. She wore protective shadings at all times when coming in direct contact with the sun and at ninety-two she had the skin of a young girl. There were few wrinkles, no pigmentary discolorations and little dryness. Granted some of her good skin had to be genetic in origin, but the care she had given her skin had rewarded her with an appearance which was indeed enviable. Obviously her skin and its care had become something of a fetish to her, and possibly a bit of a bore to her companions, but the result was a living proof of what a modified and intelligent approach to the sun and one's skin can accomplish.

In addition to protective cosmetics the person who enjoys the life in the sun should use fewer soaps and detergents in middle age and old age and use more water-in-oil and oil-in-water emulsions (cold creams, vanishing creams) to counteract sun drying. The use of sunbathing oils *after* exposure is frequently as effective as before or during, but one should remember that external oils alone are of little value in restoring or preserving body moisture so essential to skin health and beauty. Additionally, the heat of the sun can cause damage. Dermatologists in the American Southwest, where skin cancer is endemic, have concluded that not only sunlight but also heat is a major factor in photosensitive skin eruptions. Patients subject to solar keratoses and sun cancer were free of these disturbances in a cool climate at 6500 feet altitude even when exposed to powerful sunlight. Again, your seasons in the sun should be regulated by your knowledge of your own skin, and by your own observation of solar effects. A word to the wise should be sufficient . . . but is it?

The identity of your skin in lore and language could be an indication of how important, subconsciously, man has always considered his skin. Before the story of skin became a medical specialty man conveyed thoughts about his skin in his everyday *patois.* You "itch" to be active; you feel like "jumping out of your skin"; you would not care to be in "Jonathan or Susie's skin"; you want to "save your own skin"; you survive by the "skin of your teeth" and you give your enemy a "hiding" or "tanning."

Skinning is cheating; *flaying* is scathing criticism. A sensitive person is "thin-skinned." People can be "rubbed the wrong way," cut to the "quick," or you can have something or someone "get under your skin."

In relation to the "something under the skin," a very famous early American surgeon in his memoirs tells of operating on a slave (the story is pre-Civil War) who had a severe twitching nerve in her lower thigh muscles which needed to be severed. The old woman had become convinced a lizard had jumped up her skirt and gotten under her skin. So great was her conviction that the doctor knew he had to produce the lizard. An ardent fundamentalist Presbyterian, the doctor agonized over the dilemma of sending his sons (who were determined also to become doctors) in search of a lizard to produce and have them witness a lie, or to have his operation prove useless unless his patient could behold the lizard, extracted from "under her skin" by the doctor's magical scalpel. His oath to Hippocrates prevailed and the good Christian doctor cured his patient and I suppose rationalized his medical untruth to his sons.

Primitive people literally identified the skin with the individual, prized the skins of their foes as trophies of war. Medieval English villagers nailed the skins of raiding Danes to the church door. Victorian jewelry was often made of the skin of one's ancestors' hair braided intricately into the form of a necklace. One of the more prized style of "engagement" rings was a gold finger ring with a lock of the beloved's hair (an appendage of the skin) curled artistically beneath a medallion of cut glass.

As recently as our own generation, a sinister use of skin was evidenced in Nazi Germany with the famous lamps executed by Ilse Koch from the skin of the interned and deceased Jewish inhabitants of the camp at Buchenwald. Incredibly some of these relics of modern day barbarism are still exhibited. Some macabre by-paths of medical interest in the skin are these anthropodermic oddities: Sir William Harvey, the father of our knowledge of the circulatory system, presented a tanned human hide to the College of Physicians in London; Hermann Boerhaave's famed Leyden Surgical Museum exhibited three complete human skins and a pair of high-heeled lady's shoes made of the epidermis of an executed criminal; royal surgeon Pierre Sue, father of the novelist Eugene, presented to the Cabinet de Roi a pair of human skin leather slippers. Prized by a caretaker at Edinburgh University was a wallet made of the skin of William Burke, the celebrated corpse purveyor, and physicians even as late as the twentieth century have been known to carry anthropodermic wallets and cigarette cases as mementos of their student days in the dissecting room. Other anthropodermic treasures were belts, suspenders, book bindings, especially of erotica, and court records of a murderer's trial bound in his own skin.

The greatest anthropodermic skin scandal before Ilse Koch's lamps was an 1883 Tewkesbury case against an almshouse trustee for selling deceased inmates' skins to the New England shoe industry. This caused a national scandal but was never proven to be fact.

The belief that an individual's personality lives on in his skin after death seems to be inherent in all cultures. Possibly the greatest opposition to cremation after death is this idea, compounded with the individual's innate fear of death by burning. Famous in the stories of an individual's survival through his skin after death is the story of the drum made of the skin of Frederick the Great's fearsome General Ziska. After his death, the drumbeat was still heard. While alive the general terrified his foes with the beat of his drum.

Two Nobel prize winners in fiction, William Faulkner and Ernest Hemingway, created short stories in which preservation of skin after death plays the leading role. In Faulkner's story the heroine lived and slept for years at the bedside of her dead lover in a psychotic denial that he did not continue to live in the dead skin hanging to his skeleton; in Hemingway's a mountain climber high in the Alps hung his lantern, from expediency, on the jaw of his dead wife's unburied corpse. In both stories, the dead person continued to live even though the skin had crackled and degenerated because the skin was the true casket of the inner person to the two individuals who were left behind to dispose of the remains.

Interestingly enough the anthropodermic idiosyncrasies of man do not appear to be any more offensive to the animal lover than man's common use of the skin and flesh of other animals. The true vegetarian, for example, is just as repelled by the sight of alligator or snake skin shoes, mink, fox, leopard and other animal skin coats and rugs as he is by the taste of the flesh of the animal used for food purposes. So intense is the current interest in the survival of the species on this planet that the lady who once shunned the wearing of a fake fur, or the use of a fake fur on her floor or in her pillows, is today the sponsor of the synthetic fabrics which create the illusion, rather than using the original pelts. Our current interest in skin extends beyond our own to that of our animal companions.

To many African and Melanesian peoples the skin is the

source of human immortality. Men die when they have lost the power to shed their skins. And to a great extent, as we shall see, there is some scientific truth in their beliefs.

The most primitive of our emotions are revealed in our skin. Fear shows in the pallor; anxiety or embarrassment in the flush; fright and relief in the sweating. It is a well-known fact that lawyers often depend upon the ability of the client's skin reflections to convince a jury when the client is under duress. To maintain a "cool" is a large part of today's human success. The individual caught in a lie often reveals it by a sudden flush, a sweat or a ghostly white cloud passing across the face. The dramatist and the novelist have used these skin manifestations in order to convey to the reader the inner emotions of the character. In life we become accustomed, consciously or unconsciously, to judging the human behaviour by external changes in the skin.

These skin responses are maintained during sleep as well as when you are awake. Released from cortical inhibitions civilized man rubs and scratches himself with animal abandon under the direction of his lower brain centers. One of my patients, a highly intelligent individual, was coping with an external skin affliction caused by an allergy to sand fleas. The condition could be kept under control, as the patient was quite capable of not scratching as long as she was conscious of the workings of her mind and subsequent behaviour. But when she slept and the irritation pursued, she resorted to the relief of itching by scratching. The only solution to the problem was to tie her hands in mittens, cover her disturbed skin areas with bandages and plastic occlusive dressings, and keep her reasonably sedated during sleep until the skin had been given sufficient time and peace to heal.

Naturally, since strong emotions reflect their images on the skin it is logical to understand that these same emotions, when suppressed in the conscious cerebral areas, find quick and often violent expression in the outer skin. That is why, today, in the age of the "cool," your dermatologist is concerned with the effects of suppressed anger, frustration, hostility, resentment upon your outer skin in forms of skin diseases and the cures which have become increasingly more important than the mere application of salves and creams to the surface skin. Lotions, potions, and pomades will not alone suffice. The cures in many cases have been effected through hypnosis, psychiatric consultation and eventual readjustment to emotional disorders which seem to be controlled by the individual, while the skin of that person is evidencing his inner pains and anxieties.

ESTHETICS OF THE SKIN

I have a patient, conventionally bred, who was visiting in Copenhagen and guest at a private swimming, golf and tennis club when a man with a completely tattooed body (at least all that was visible to the staring pair of human eyes) poised himself upon the diving board and prepared to leap into the pool. At the moment of his appearance on the diving board everyone at the poolside rose. Much to my patient's surprise she learned that the man was none other than the King of Denmark, who was world renowned for his tattooes. Previously she had thought such "freaks" were confined to the ranks of Ringling Brothers Barnum and Bailey Circus, and never found in the exculsive realm of royalty.

Like many people my patient was unaware that tattooing, scarifications and body painting are all ancient in tradition and indicative to the anthropologist that man employed his skin before the walls of his cave for means of communication with his fellow man.

Tattooing—the most commonplace esthetic usage of the skin, has been occupied for sundry purposes: for warding off evil spirits; for bringing good luck; for adding sexual allure; for identification (in Hitler's Germany the ill-fated Jews were labelled and catalogued with the sign of the Star of David and a serial number); for medical purposes in checking a key point of the body for reference. It has been practical in the space program in marking our astronauts for the attachment of vital instruments to their bodies. And, it highlighted one of the most successful commercial advertising campaigns in publication history—the Marlboro man with his tattooed hand, lighting his favorite cigarette. That man became the symbol of the rugged, all-American, outdoor male whose tattoo indicated a mysterious past of adventure and sophistication concealed beneath his pure, wholesome, male image.

Tattooing has known many vogues. It has been "in" and it has been "out." Currently among the hippie-culture-oriented youth it is "in," and used by both sexes to convey upon their bodies the message of love—and peace. Yet, almost daily, your dermatologist is confronted with a patient who wishes to have a tattoo removed. On the patient's body (usually the forearm, hand or chest) is the tattooed story of entrapment with another human being, someone removed from the person the patient is now living with. Such a memento of a past romance must be obliterated. The tattoo has to go—or the new romance will be gone.

That tattoo, written on the skin in a moment of madness or intoxication—physical or romantic—does not have to remain with you until death you doth part. It can be removed. The methods of removal are many, but the most successful and pleasing cosmetic results are achieved by superficial abrasion of the skin.

It was in Puerto Rico that I first learned of the removal of tattoos with the application of ordinary table salt. One rubs the skin until it becomes bright red in the tattooed area of the skin. The procedure is repeated about twice during the next six months, and in many cases the tattoo is completely removed. (It might be of interest to know that the superstitious in Puerto Rico only use the table salt technique in the light of the full moon!)

Today, this simple method has been medically refined and is applied in your doctor's office. It is a technique known as *salabrasion.* It is an easily controlled method in which a very mild dermabrasion of uniform depth may be accomplished. (For further details see the section on dermabrasion.)

The relatively moderate manner in which the abrasion is accomplished contributes to a large extent in the good results once the tattoo is removed. The gentleness of salabrasion is evident if the skin is examined immediately following the treatment, when one may observe some of the vellus hairs within the area still unbroken.

In salabrasion no freezing of the skin is required, as the salt itself is somewhat anesthetic. Most of the discomfort results from the pressure of the rubbing. Even so, this irritation cannot begin to equal the original pain of having the tattoo applied. However, one should realize that most tattooes are done in a tattoo parlor when one is in a festive, carefree carnival spirit—usually "stoned" or at least somewhat inebriated or high.

The first few days following the salabrasion, there is little change and two or three visits to your doctor are required. I might add as a word of forewarning that, despite the simplicity of the Puerto Rican salt remedy for removing tattooes, I would not endorse it or recommend it as a "home remedy,"—under full moon, or quarter! If you have a tattoo which you wish to banish from your sight, consult an expert. In the final analysis, this is much less complicated.

To understand man's desire to tattoo his body one must recognize that the art is an old and accomplished one. As early as the fourteenth century B.C. the heretic Pharaoh, Ikhnaton, and his queen of great beauty, Nefertete, submitted to the tattooist's needle to record on their breasts and arms some hieroglyphics of their God, Aton, who was new and controversial. And, the reddish coloring of the ochre on skeletal remains uncovered in prehistoric sites indicates that Ice Age inhabitants painted the skin of corpses, possibly in a primitive attempt to restore life by simulating the color of the blood of the living.

Tattooing reached its culmination as an art form among the Marquesans, who appeared to the first Europeans to follow Captain Cook's original expeditions in the eighteenth century. They seemed to be wearing exotically patterned tights, since the tattoos covered every inch of their bodies from hairline to foot. Patterns were continued on eyelids, nostrils, soles of the hands and feet and sometimes even the tongue. Many were the same designs carved and painted on their famed canoes. The building of the Marquesan canoe was an "affair of religion" and the *kahuna,* the canoe building expert, had transcribed upon his face and body the designs and motifs of the canoes whose construction he had supervised. The designs were different for men and women—delicate and elusive for the women in contrast to solid, powerful motifs adopted by the men. Marquesan "patu-tiki" (tattooing) depicted crabs, tortoises and lizards, and they fitted into geometric designs which were bold and strong on the arms and legs, and delicate as they centered about the extremeties with the hands of the women looking as if they were encased in fine Irish-lace mittens. It is generally believed that the human-looking motifs represented evil spirits.

Being a dermatologist and located in the South Pacific during the Korean War with the Air Force, I became especially interested in the tattoos, their history and their esthetic appeal as a form of art. In New Zealand, for example, the Maori devoted their talents to preserving the more reliable and unmistakable tattoos of their ancestors. Originally, the Maori preserved and tattooed the heads of family and friends as relics to be wept over on appropriate occasions of mourning or ancestor-worship. This custom of baking tattooed portraits on original heads led eventually to a gruesome trade between the native chieftains and foreign curio collectors. As the demands for the preserved heads became greater among the British agents and visiting ships, it became dangerous to continue preparing family heads that might eventually fall into foreign or enemy hands. In the American Museum of Natural History one can see some fine examples of desiccated Maori trophy heads, tattooed with the intricate *moko* facial tattoo which was the pride of a Maori warrior. The tattoos of the Maori nobles were derived from carved wood designs and created by albatross bone needles dipped into soot to create the bluish patterns which emphasized the face structure. These funerary portraits are, now very rare and considered as art trophies, treasured by private museums and individual collectors.

In Japan, where tattooing reached a fine art and where many English and American sailors obtained their original tattoos, the tattoo had its purpose in preserving and disseminating items of national interest and folklore. Before printing facilities were available through the means of the printing presses, the Japanese tattooed his body with historical data and legend. Elaborately tattooed on the bodies of the famous foot-runners were illustrations of treasured legends which were passed from province to province and made known for several generations until they were incorporated into a formalized written form of preservation. The more familiar style of Japanese tattooing was not unlike their art form—composed of faces, flower arrangements, delicately posed figures of the stylized No and Kabuki dancers and the ever-present demon and dragon. It was also in Japan that tattoos were originally used to brand criminals. And in the Orient, the telltale tattoo was a means of introduction to the drug dealer, or the individual who participated in the white slave traffic.

As the Polynesian skin tattoo moved westward from the South Seas, we find similar bird and beast designs removed to the totem poles of the Haidi Indians in the Northwest and tattooed on their bodies for decorative designs. The Indian designs are almost abstract in their formal, bifurcated tattoos. Later we find the tattoo replaced with animal motifs painted temporarily on the human skin, especially on the face, to emulate the qualities associated with a revered animalistic ancestor of their totemistic religion. Stylized motifs include their paintings of whole animals or characteristic parts intended to invoke envied attributes of strength or acumen. A wolf head or foot, an eagle beak or wing, the silhouette of the killer whale, these were painted as bold emblems, sweeping obliquely across the face, often crossing one eye, one cheek or a part of the chin. Or the design might cover only the eye and chin areas.

Among other North American Indian tribes face painting was used as a sign of mood. The design might indicate the warrior was in love, melancholy, or simply busy trapping (this latter he indicated by a zig-zag on his soot-blackened face). In the Indian ritual dances we see a panorama of the fact that the Indian's inner urge to communicate and express his artistic, creative self was indeed more than skin deep.

In Africa—the tribes dwelling on the Gold Coast, the Ivory Coast and in certain sections of the Congo—men's skin was embellished with scarifications. In contrast to the smooth Polynesian tattooing, the cicatrix is raised above the level of the skin. These geometric scarifications served as heraldic designs designating tribe, district and sometimes rank.

The scarification of the women is especially important in these countries. It begins when the girl has just learned to walk and continues at least until puberty with the other women in the tribe doing the art work. The motifs include stripings, looped designs and, among the Bangonga, concentric circles. The African tribesmen attest to the erotic potency of cicatrices raised on their mates' upper arms, buttocks and in the pubic areas. They find them beautiful, provocative, exciting and fully believe that they accentuate movements of sexual contact. This is possibly true: the early invasion of those areas strengthens the girl and eliminates her early fears of sexual violation. As it is ritualistic and a culturally accepted part of the eventual sexual expression, scarification probably does psychologically tend to induce sexual potency.

The proof of scarification and tattooing as vital rites in the early African civilizations comes from the surface patterns notable on several different types of African sculpture. There are some beautiful portrait heads, discovered as late as 1938. These heads were cut from life and cast in brass. The heads are incredibly realistic, combining Hamitic and Mongolian traits along with the Negroid. These heads are scarred with vertical striations of an eighth of an inch apart, covering the entire face including the eyelids and sometimes the lower lip. (Incidentally, in many cultures we find the color tattooing of the lips not uncommon before the discovery of satisfactory lip rouges of wax.)

Since the Old Testament enjoined the Israelites against the practice of tattooing, it was forbidden by Mohammed, and a Roman Catholic Council condemned the "marking of the skin with punctures accentuated by pigment," tattooing in Western cultures has been somewhat tabu. It was introduced to Europe and America by seamen who visited faraway places. The tattoo was almost the insignia of the wandering male who roamed the universe and became a member of the international fraternity of adventurous spirits who were not immune to the thoughts and habits of men living in other cultures. The writings of Robert Louis Stevenson, W. H. Hudson and Herman Melville were of heroes who broke with the rigidity of custom in Europe and America and became linked to the unknown, the primitive, the adventurous. The tattoo was their emblem. The individual who preferred the comforts of his home, the possession of a Gauguin extolling the beauty of the Polynesian, the reading of an adventure story, had little in common with the sailor who sailed the seven seas and returned home with his body tattooed in remembrance of the things past. For years the tattoo separated the "gentleman" from the bum, but as travel and war brought man closer together, the understanding and appreciation of the legendary tattoos has increased. Today the tattoo can belong to a king, or a wandering alienated man using his skin for a means of communication and identification.

The painting of the skin of the face, like tattooing, is as old, almost, as man himself—and as contemporary as the beauty salons of Elizabeth Arden. The red ochre used in the burial rituals, the blue woad of the ancient Britons, the kohl utilized in Asia to enhance eye beauty have all filtered into the melting pots of the leading cosmeticians who have utilized them to suit the demands of current fashion trends. The highly decorated eyes of today, complete with false eyelashes, would have been scorned a generation ago, just as the painted fingernails which were once the trademark of "ladies of the evening" are now commonplace and the "Does she or doesn't she?" question in hair dye is so accepted that it is taken for granted that "she does." Today, our current vogue is for the "natural look" but we resort to a lot of subterfuge to achieve that "natural look." Fashion is fickle and fleeting and whatever the "look" might be, it is completely fashion's whim. The fact cannot be better illustrated than in an article which appeared in "The Spectator" written by Joseph Addison (1672 to 1719). It pertains to the use of *patches,* an obsolete form of a skin esthetic in today's school of fashion:

> About the middle of last winter, I went to see an opera at the Theatre in the Haymarket, where I could not but take notice of two parties of very fine women that had placed themselves in the opposite side boxes,

and seemed drawn up in a kind of battle array one against another. After a short survey of them, I found they were "patched" differently; the faces on one hand being spotted on the right side of the forehead, and those upon the other on the left. I quickly perceived that they cast hostile glances upon one another and that their patches were placed in those different situations, as party signals to distinguish friends from foes. In the middle boxes between these two opposite bodies were several ladies who patched indifferently on both sides of their faces, and seemed to sit there with no other intention but to see the opera. Upon my inquiry, I found that the body of Amazons on my right hand were Whigs; and those on my left, Tories; and that those who placed themselves in the middle boxes were a neutral party, whose faces had not yet declared themselves. These last as I afterwards found, diminished daily, and took their party with one side or the other; insomuch that I observed in several of them, the patches which were before dispersed equally, are now all gone over to the Whig or Tory side of the face. The censorious say that the men whose hearts are aimed at are very often the occasions that one side of the face is thus dishonored, and lies under a kind of disgrace, while the other is so much set off and adorned by the owner; and that the patches turn to the right or the left, according to the principles of the man who is most in favor. But whatever may be the motives of the few fantastical coquets, who do not patch for the public good, so much as for their own private advantage it is certain there are several women of honour who patch out of principle and with an eye to their country. Nay, I am informed that some of them adhere so steadfastly to their party, and are so far from sacrificing their zeal for the public to their passion for any particular person, that in a late draught of marriage articles a lady has stipulated with her husband that whatever his opinions are, she shall be at liberty to patch on which side she pleases.

I am told that many virtuous matrons, who formerly have been taught to believe that this artificial spotting of the face was unlawful are now reconciled by a zeal for their cause, to what they could not be prompted by a concern for their beauty. This way of declaring war upon one another puts me in mind of what is reported of the tigress, that several spots rise in her skin when she is angry; or as Mr. Cowley has imitated the verses that stand as the motto of this paper,

> "She swells with angry pride,
> And calls forth all her spots on every side."

When I was in the theatre the time above mentioned, I had the curiosity to count the patches on both sides, and found the Tory patches to be about twenty stronger than the Whig; but to make amends for this small inequality, I the next morning found the whole puppet show filled with faces spotted after the Whiggish manner. Whether or not the ladies had retreated hither in order to rally their forces I cannot tell; but the next night they came in so great a body to the opera that they outnumbered the enemy.

This account of part patches will, I am afraid, appear improbable to those who live at a distance from the fashionable world; but as a distinction it is a distinction of a very singular nature, and what perhaps might never meet with a parallel, I think I should not have discharged the office of a faithful spectator had I not recorded it."

—From "The Spectator" No. 81

So reader be cautious. Your politically minded friend might be identified with a patch on either the left or the right side of the cheek, or an identifying tattoo on the wrist. Your skin has served such a purpose before. Nothing in skin decor is new or especially unique. From the stretching of the lips of the Ubangi to the piercing of the ears of girl babies for earrings (believed in some locales to be a sign of good luck, in others as assuring eye strength) skin has been and will continue to be a sign of the inner psyche. You may embellish it with messages of love or hate, mutilate it with symbols of class identity, or deploy it to convey messages of intrigue—amorous or political. But whatever you do as a sign of the times, you are merely using your skin to convey some of the frustrations you are unable to vocalize. Just remember it is not irrevocable.

THE NEEDS OF YOUR SKIN

In one circle there is a medical philosophy which indicates that from the moment of birth, the process leading ultimately to death sets in.

Modern geriatrics has altered, somewhat, this school of thinking. The exact date when physical deterioration sets in is not yet determined, but it is not necessarily regarded as the process of—"with life, death ensues." Some doctors believe the age to be about twenty-one, others place it younger (puberty to be exact), while still another school has it commencing after thirty-five or following the decline of the endocrine glands, the traditional change-of-life period. At this moment of writing there has been no date fixed. But, we do know that there is a degenerative process of age which affects different people at different ages and stages of life.

As we have said, your skin is basically genetic in form and whatever the pattern of your forebearers was in relation to aging will be your pattern also. With this foreknowledge there still are certain procedures which you can utilize (this side of plastic surgery) which will help give longer life to your skin and generally affect your physical appearance. Amazingly, most of the procedures are quite simple in origin and application. The number one consideration beyond your heritage is the recognition of the fact that your skin reflects your inner being. If you are in generally good health with all of your systems functioning properly you will usually radiate this state of health with the fresh, lusty complexion which is a barometer of general good health. To obtain this appearance, people have gone through all manner of behavior from faddish diets to the reading of good thoughts to culminate in the essential truth . . . "I think, therefore, I am," or as has been conversely stated, "I am, therefore, I think." This was a popular practice in the nineteenth century especially among pregnant women who seriously believed if they thought good thoughts, read good literature, studied good art, the fetus growing within them would be visibly affected and emerge a creation of total beauty. Today, we know there is very little scientific reasoning in this process, but we do admit that the skin mirrors the general physical condition of the inner body and as I have previously stated it often indicates to the professional eye a serious disease which has not yet given outwardly any acute manifestations. People have often observed that a young woman in the second trimester of pregnancy will reach the epitome of feminine beauty because all of her glands are functioning properly, nature has adjusted her to her condition and she is totally relaxed. She is, actually, living for the fetus growing within her and in the process glows with an inner radiance that is a combination of the physical and the spiritual.

Realistically, there is not much compensation in the thoughts of Sir Thomas More that although youth gave us "love and roses, age leaves us with wine and friends . . ." In a youth-oriented culture such as we know today, the illusion of youth is very important and over and above all physical manifestations of youth, your skin is the telltale denominator. How then do we care for and protect this enormous organ which encloses all of our inner being?

One, we start with birth and an understanding of the logical degenerative forces which will in time leave their mark. When you are born your skin averages 387.5 square inches in size and when you have reached the adult stage it has increased to approximately 2786.4 square inches. The surface area from birth to maturity undergoes a seven-fold increase. Your body weight meanwhile increases about twenty-fold.

The capacity of your skin to move and be stretched depends on its own thickness, the number of its folds, its intrinsic elasticity, firmness of fixation by the *tela subcutanea* (a cobweb-like structure), and the age of the individual. The weight of your skin is about 16 percent of your body weight. In men, skin weighs about 10½ pounds and in women about seven pounds. The subcutaneous fat weighs about twenty-six pounds in men and about thirty-three in women. The specific gravity of skin is about 1.25.

The skin of the abdomen has the greatest capacity for extension, but when it is extended beyond its capacity (as in a woman during pregnancy) the skin becomes permanently damaged. The pregnancy scars *(striae gravidarum)* appear during pregnancy as red streaks but after the baby is born they become permanent white lines called *lineae albicantes.*

The same type of lines can appear on the body after the loss of excessive fat or swelling.

The differentiation in the embryonic cleavages and the furrows one is born with—those lines of your skin which stretch over the years—is slight and basically environmental in origin.

Once the fetus has emerged from the liquid of the womb and become a human being, the embryonic cleavages begin to alter to the ultimate identity of the life lines.

These lines, evidenced in the foot and palm of the new-born babe, are clearly defined at the moment of birth and they are lines which, although they enlarge proportionately with maturity, are the life lines at the hour of death. It was through the study of these furrows that Sir Francis Galton established the science of fingerprinting for identification.

Shakespeare classically explained man's life lines from infancy to senility in Jaques "seven stages of life" soliloquy from *As You Like It:* "At first, the infant, mewling and puking in the nurse's arms," and at the last, ". . . second childishness and mere oblivion, sans teeth, sans eyes, sans taste, sans everything." In the familiar Kersh photograph of Sir Winston Churchill we see elucidated the resemblance between the wrinkled, frowning, hairless babe and the growling, furrowed, balding old man.

Due to the elasticity of the individual life lines with which you are born, surgeons, when operating, make their incisions (when possible) parallel to these lines rather than crosswise where the tension is (naturally) greater and the healing process more difficult.

Since nutrition is important to skin beauty, for centuries the quest for skin beauty "fad" diets has appeared and reappeared. For example, Egyptians periodically fasted and took purgatives to maintain the slim, sinewy, square shouldered, flat bellied, high pelviced creature we know from the bas-reliefs and murals. To improve their complexions they had a habit of eating dried figs three times a day for a period of seven days. Hippocrates, the father of medicine, recommended a diet for perfect skin which consisted of barley roll dipped in wine for breakfast, salt fish, ham, bread, and wine for lunch and fish or beef with wine, vegetables, and fruit for dinner.

Most diets are based upon a discovery more than a century ago by an English doctor, R. P. Banting, who postulated that it was not the amount of food which caused weight increase, but the amount of carbohydrates. Since this discovery most diets have been protein, some fat, and non-alcoholic beverages. However the "scotch-and-steak" or "bourbon-and-beef" Madison Avenue Drinking Man's Diets are contradictory to most subscribed formulas for dieting. These diets are based upon the familiar biochemical formula that carbohydrates burn in the flame of the fats. In short, you burn up your own fat with a Steak Tartare and a bottle of bourbon. However, any diet can have side effects upon certain individuals (the high protein one often causes extreme diarrhea, for example) and no diet should be entered into without first consulting a physician and seeing if the cause of your overweight is something more than "over-indulgence." A thyroid dysfunction could exist and the loss of food will only make you have less energy and a loss of weight will not ensue.

Certain vitamin supplements are advisable for different skin conditions, all of which are customarily prescribed by the attendant physician, for example Vitamin B for shingles;

Vitamin A for acne (in addition to a restrictive diet regarding certain sweets and butter fats); Vitamin K for abnormal bruising.

The ladies of Rome dieted to keep their Aphrodite- or Venus-like figures and were infatuated with the idea of aphrodisiacs. Male gonads were reputedly used as youth rejuvenators and aphrodisiacs. In the Middle Ages, wrinkles and skin blemishes were supposedly eliminated by the eating of garlic and the distilled juice of beans. The virgin white beauty of the pre-Renaissance women was sought in a diet of gravel, ashes and tallow. And, in the eighteenth century women attempted to achieve the same effects by swallowing mercury or drinking spring water containing arsenic. Through the centuries, diets have run the gamut and no matter what diet you and your contemporaries have hit upon, it has been thought of before. As has been said, there is "no new thing under the sun." (*Ecclesiates,* 1:9)

HOW DO YOU CARE FOR YOUR SKIN?

In truth, the simplest remedy for care of the skin is *water.* Yet even excessive bathing can be harmful and bathing with injurious water can produce dermatitis. The difference between *hard* and *soft* water is important, especially in your cosmetics. Hard water, for instance, contains a large quantity of dissolved and undissolved salts which render soap largely insoluble and make it unsuitable for washing. The quality of water which varies from city to city creates many skin problems for people when moving from one environment to another, until they adjust or discover a catalyst which will make the water usable. Soft water, which is rain water or fresh water, should be used whenever possible. People who live in the Virgin Islands, for example, having transferred from the continent, are amazed to discover the difference in their skin and hair textures when living in the islands where all water is stored rain water.

Hard water can be softened by boiling or adding borax, washing soda, or glycerine to the washing water.

Aside from washing, water in the form of steam, poultices, compresses and medicinal baths, is also used to soften, warm or cool the skin. Water is also used as a solvent in the bases of medicines, and face and hair lotions. And most of the creams employed for cosmetic purposes are contingent upon the use of water.

The best cleanser of the skin is *soap.* Soap is made by boiling fats with alkalies. Soaps fall into two categories, hard—made with sodium hydroxide (lye or soda ash)—is known as *soda soap;* soft (ointment) soap made with potassium hydroxide is *potash or green soap.* If your soap is strongly alkaline it will make your skin slippery. When household soap and commercial detergents are used in warm water or when the lather of green soap is allowed to remain and dry on the skin, both will cause desquamation (a scaling and peeling) and a dermatitis can set in if either is used too often—thus the phrase *dishpan hands.*

Many dermatologists recommend Neutrogena soap for both skin and hair. The skin soap is clear, the solid shampoo soap is green. Both are hypo-allergenic. For skins that cannot use soap, there are soap substitutes available. Lowila cake is very good.

Alcohol is used by dermatologists for treatment as a vigorous disinfecting chemical and for drying and grease dissolving. Eau de cologne is an alcoholic solution of various essential oils and can be used for drying as can the face astringents which often have added ingredients of camphor, and menthol for cooling purposes. Tincture of benzoin is a common ingredient in astringents as are acetic acid and witch hazel. To produce the same effects, for example when washing one's hair, vinegar or fresh lemon juice added to the rinsing water will neutralize the irritating alkaline of the soap and, in addition, add lustre to your hair.

Ointments, salves and creams are used extensively in cosmetics—either alone or as a basis carrying remedial agents for the skin. The commonplace base materials for such products are of animal, vegetable, and mineral origin.

Lanolin, the fat of wool, is perhaps the most commonly used animal ointment base material. It becomes rancid slowly. Hydrous lanolin, which is lanolin that can contain water, is the best type of lanolin used in a cleansing cream. It frequently sensitizes, however, and for those people who find lanolin too heavy (it sometimes clogs the pores), Shepard's Lotion (lanolin-free) is highly recommended as a substitute. Another agreeable and pleasant animal ointment base material is white wax but it turns rancid quickly. Goose fat, fresh lard and butter are used in lipsticks.

Favorite vegetable ointment base materials are olive oil, sesame oil, sweet almond oil and castor oil for keratoses and sunburn. Cocoa butter is much used (it is a basic ingredient for some of the more popular sun-tan lotions), but it is a solid and unless scented carries a strong odor. For your own "do it yourself" cosmetic kit, you may use any of the vegetable oils alone or together with one of the mentioned astringent properties, and prepare your own emollient to cleanse and soften your skin. Solid Crisco, a highly refined preparation of cottonseed oil, is an excellent lubricant—odorless, free from becoming rancid, and non-sensitizing.

Vaseline is the most commonplace mineral oil used in cosmetics. It is produced from petroleum and must be absolutely purified before applying to your skin. Incidentally, American white vaseline is world famous because it is absolutely free from petroleum and the sulphuric acid found in the yellow vaseline used for medicinal dressings.

Solid paraffin and paraffin oil are also popular ingredients found in cosmetic creams. For years the inserting of paraffin under the skin was a commonplace practice, especially among people in the theatre. The story is told of the famous actor playing Hamlet behind the heated gas footlights of a nineteenth century theater. When he reached the famous line: "O, that this too, too solid flesh would melt, thaw, resolve itself into a dew . . ." the words became actuality as the paraffin in his cheeks began to dissolve visibly and age took over the paraffin injected face. Paraffin was also used as a breast uplift until the recent popularity of silicone.

When I first entered the practice of dermatology I had an elderly lady patient who was grotesquely deformed by the presence of huge tumors on her cheeks, neck and breasts. The tumors were caused by injections of paraffin. My patient revealed that she had been a star performer in one of the large circuses for many years and was obliged as a trapeze artist to keep her weight at approximately ninety pounds. In order not to appear to be aging or hungrily gaunt she was obliged to have paraffin injections in her cheeks, neck and breasts. The presence of these foreign objects in her skin tissues had caused the tumor formations. The prognosis was negative as the tumors continued to recur after surgery. Quite a few *paraffinomata* were seen following its extensive usage in the nineteenth and early twentieth century. The problems which silicone injections might cause have not yet begun to appear in drastic numbers as the procedure is reasonably new for diagnosis or prediction regarding the eventual results in the sex-goddesses of the sixties and seventies.

Glycerine may be used in place of fats. It is very compatible with alcohol and water and the old fashion glycerin and rose water is still a favorite with many people. Pure glycerin can be applied to a well moistened skin or a solution can be made of fifty percent glycerine and water. Ten or fifteen percent glycerin can be added to astringents to ward off the drying effect, and before applying the popular pancake make-up your skin can be protected and moistened with a cleansing of glycerin and water.

The type of cream or cleansing you choose for your skin is contingent upon the type of skin you are born with. A dry skin must be protected against everything which makes it dry: soap, alcohol, benzene, hot steam, cold water, wind and sun. And it should be greased several times a day with a soothing cream, the excess of which is wiped off with a soft cloth. It is advisable to have greasy massages once or twice a week with warm oil treatments afterwards. If the skin is less dry you may at rare intervals allow lukewarm water and super-fatted soap (*e.g.* Basis, Oilatum or Emulave. Pear's glycerine is an excellent soap) but after washing the face it must be smeared with cream. The cream should be allowed to remain on the skin until all or a great part has been absorbed and should be removed with a glycerin-and-water cleanser.

Oily and rough skin can be helped by the use of such soaps as Fels Naphtha or even the abrasive Lava soap, provided the skin is not infected or inflamed and irritated. Simple astringents such as witch hazel and rubbing alcohol also aid in removing the excess oil. Soy-Dome cleanser is an excellent and soothing soybean preparation to be used on irritated or sensitive skin.

By the care of your skin I mean the systematic treatment of the healthy skin and the underlying tissues, with the aim of keeping both fresh and healthy as long as possible. It was Seneca who said hundreds of years ago, "We don't die, we commit suicide." Your skin is an outward mask of your suicidal intent. The means of skin care at your disposal are: increasing your blood circulation, enhancing the elasticity of the blood vessels in the skin; increasing muscle tension; keeping the sebaceous ducts always clean (a most imperative act during adolescence); drying the greasy skin, and oiling the dry skin.

In your outward appearance the skin of your face is most important and therefore I will detail some of the treatment care you can perform. Massage by hand and by machine, steam, cooled vapor, cold and warm fomentations, packs, compresses and oil treatments are methods used in the care of your face. The application of cosmetics following the care is an art which you have to study and adapt to your face and your type of looks.

MASSAGE

Never massage a face with acne impetigo or infected eczema. You might spread the infection further on the skin surface.

The proper massage is performed by a person other than yourself—preferably a trained technician who knows not to work against the muscle formation and inadvertently break the tissue, and start the aging process before nature does. Many examples of bad massage can be seen among men and women who have been patted and massaged by a bad masseur.

The massage must be given with well-greased massaging hands. *First,* place the fingers of both hands in the middle of the forehead and *stroke towards the temples. Second,* put the fingers of both hands on the bridge of the nose and with the entire palms make smoothing movements in the shape of a half circle towards the temples. *Third,* take the chin between the middle and ring fingers of both hands and smooth the palms towards the temples.

The most important thing in massage is to remember that the movements of the massaging hands always go up towards the temples. The approach must be gentle, lifting the chin upward and the wrinkles outward. When patting, pat with one hand until there is a sensation of stimulus and then stroke gently with the other hand. The hand massage should not last more than ten minutes.

In addition, there is massage by mechanical vibrators. The mechanical units can be purchased at any pharmaceutical house. A rubber sponge attachment is best for face use. There is one vibrator which is attached to the hand to give added stimulus when hand-massaging. The directions are the same: upward and outward on the forehead, on the face toward the ears, on the chin backward, and downward on the neck.

STEAMING THE FACE

Hot steam softens the epidermis, loosens the sebaceous plugs (blackheads) which close up the sebaceous ducts and make the plugs easier to remove. Cover your head with a thick towel so there will be little steam escaping from alongside your head. The time allotted for steaming should be from three to ten minutes.

It is inadvisable to expose a dry face to the drying effect of hot steam. If your skin is dry, hot poultices may be used to dilate the blood vessels. Cold water poultices make the skin cool and constrict the blood vessels and the openings of the sebaceous ducts. After steaming, small amounts of benzoin (available in any drug store), Eau de cologne or white vinegar can be added to a cold-water compress. Ice can also be used, but a reactive inflammation may follow the sudden constriction of your vessels.

FACE PACKS

Packs are a supplementary part of facial treatment. Packs as a beauty aid go far back in history. The ingredients used run the gamut from mud to eggs.

Mud packs, extremely popular in geographical areas where spas flourish, are marketed either as powders (Fuller's Earth), to be mixed with water, forming a paste which is spread over the face with a brush, or in tubes of cream applied with the fingers in a layer the thickness of a piece of cardboard. The drying mask makes the face feel tight and drawn. When dry (fifteen to thirty minutes) it should be washed off with luke warm water. Immediately following the treatment the skin feels velvety soft. When applying your mud pack be certain to oil the eyelids and avoid getting the mixture near the eyes.

Full body mud packs are given in certain spas but they are not advisable for use by the adventurous person who covers the body in mud, waits for the drying and then jumps into a nearby lake or sea to wash away the mud. A patient of mine did this at the insistence of some well-meaning friends and was the victim of an insidious "blister-bug" which was living in the reputedly therapeutic mud. The result was an exceedingly painful experience which blighted a well-intended holiday. Packs, to be effective, cannot be rudimentally primitive or a "back to nature" course.

Egg packs are used to restore oils to a dry face. The white of the egg is spread on the face with a brush. The egg mixture should remain on the face and neck at least fifteen, and preferably thirty, minutes. (During this period, as with all masks, the patient should be absolutely quiet and as relaxed as possible.) The mask is removed with lukewarm—almost cold—water. On a very sensitive skin the egg may cause irritation. If this happens apply olive oil soaked gauze to the skin.

Another popular facial pack is made from cooked oatmeal. After application, it is allowed to dry and then is removed with lukewarm water. Some oatmeal pack enthusiasts insist that a bit of honey mixed into the pack will give the skin an additional glow.

Warm oil packs are most desirable for very dry faces. Apply some olive oil or baby oil to your face. Cover this with a layer of gauze or tissue paper. Put a rubber mask over this layer and apply heat, with either hot towels or an electric thermophor. The pack should be gently warmed and allowed to remain from ten to fifteen minutes. (This type of pack can also be very successfully applied under a sun lamp. If this is done the eyes and the lips must be covered with cotton soaked in boric acid.) When the pack is removed, the face should be rinsed with cold water or gently rubbed with towel-wrapped ice cubes. The hot oil treatment softens the skin so the occasional comedones (blackheads) can be easily removed. Witch-hazel for an oily skin or glycerin-and-rose-water for a dry skin completes the treatment.

There are, in addition, many commercial, carbon dioxide, face packs. These contain a white powder of sodium perborate and a liquid with acetic acid. The paste is applied, and removed after it dries by rubbing it off without washing. When most of the pack has been rubbed away the remainder is removed by plenty of water. This pack has a dry, constricting effect and after the application often calls for a glycerin-type astringent.

A chemically pure paraffin, melted in a water solution, is used by dermatologists and cosmetologists on faces that are wrinkling from dryness. Using a syringe, the melted paraffin is usually sprayed onto the skin at a temperature from 140°-175° Fahrenheit. As it solidifies, the paraffin layer seals the skin hermetically. The mask is worn from ten minutes to one hour. The skin is very smooth after this treatment, (which is also used in the removing of excessive hairs). If the skin is blemished, the paraffin must be treated with appropriate drugs before applying. *This is not a "do-it-yourself" remedy.*

Systematic care is essential to healthy skin. Give yourself a treatment once or twice a week, after choosing a type suitable for *your* complexion. The following are *weekly* formulas, developed for various skin textures.

Formula for a dry complexion without blackheads:

1. Cleanse skin with a greasy cream.
2. Apply hot compresses.

3. Massage the face with the hand or an electric vibrator.
4. Apply a warm oil treatment.
5. Apply cooled vapor.
6. Apply astringent compress.
7. Apply day, vanishing, or protective cream or glycerin.
8. Apply powder and facial make-up.

Formula for a dry complexion with blackheads:

1. Cleanse with a greasy cream.
2. Massage with a greasy absorbent cream.
3. Moisten face with hot steam for three to five minutes.
4. Gently remove blackheads with cleansed fingers.
5. Apply a face pack—either egg or carbon dioxide.
6. Give face a thorough washing.
7. Apply day, vanishing cream or glycerin for base.
8. Apply light powder base for make-up.

Formula for a greasy complexion with a few blackheads but no acne lesions:

1. Cleanse the face with a soap or face lotion.
2. Give face a hand massage (without cream).
3. Moisten face with hot steam for ten to fifteen minutes.
4. Gently remove blackheads.
5. Wash the face with a constricting astringent.
6. Apply a carbon dioxide face pack.
7. Wash the face in lukewarm water.
8. Apply day cream and powder base.

Formula for a greasy complexion with many blackheads but no acne lesions:

1. Cleanse face thoroughly with face lotion.
2. Apply hot steam for ten to fifteen minutes.
3. Gently remove blackheads.
4. Massage the face with either the hand or an electric vibrator.
5. Wash the face carefully with an astringent lotion.
6. Apply a carbon dioxide face pack.
7. Give the face a thorough washing in lukewarm water.
8. Apply a day or vanishing cream.
9. Apply light powder and final make-up.

Formula for a greasy complexion with acne lesions:

1. Cleanse the face with a cleansing lotion.
2. Moisten the face with hot steam.
3. Gently remove the blackheads.
4. Wash the face with an astringent which is highly alcoholic.
5. Apply a carbon dioxide face pack for a full half hour.
6. Give the face a thorough washing with a prescribed or pharmaceutical soap.
7. Apply vanishing cream.
8. Apply dry powder and final make-up.

Writings on beautiful skin are manifold. One of the most

interesting treatises, written by the famous Spanish beauty Lola Montéz, is *The Arts of Beauty* (1818-1861).

The most perfect form will avail a woman little, unless it possesses also that *brightness* which is the finishing touch and final polish of a beautiful lady. What avails a plump and well-rounded neck or shoulder if it is dim and dingy withal? What charm can be found in the finest modelled arm if its skin is coarse and rusty? A *greater* even though molded in the shape of the most charming female arm would possess small attractions to a man of taste and refinement.

I have to tell you, ladies—and the same must be said to the gentlemen, too, that the secret of acquiring a bright and beautiful skin lies in three simple things as I have said in my lecture on Beautiful Women—temperance, exercise and cleanliness. A young lady were she as fair as Hebe, as charming as Venus herself, would soon destroy it all by too high living and late hours. Take the ordinary fare of a fashionable woman, and you have a style of living which is sufficient to destroy the greatest beauty. It is not the *quantity* so much as the *quality* of the dishes that produces the mischief. Take, for instance, only strong coffee and hot bread and butter and you have a diet which would be most destructive to beauty. The heated grease, long indulged in, is sure to derange the stomach, and, by increasing our bilious disorders, gradually overspreads the fair skin with a wan or yellow hue. After this meal comes the long fast from nine in the morning until five or six in the evening when dinner is served and the half famished beauty sits down

> to sate a keen appetite with peppered soups, fish, roast, boiled and fried meat; game, tarts, sweet-meats, ices, fruits, etc., etc., etc. How must the constitution suffer to digest the *melange!* How does the healthy complexion bear witness to the combustion within? Let the fashionable lady keep up this habit and add the other of late hours and her own looking glass will tell her "we all do fade as the leaf." The firm texture of the rounded form gives way to a flabby softness or yields to a scraggy leanness, or shapeless fate. The once fair skin assumes a pallid rigidity or bloated redness which the deluded victim would still regard as the roses of health and beauty. And, when she at last becomes aware of her condition to repair the ravages she flies to paddings to give shape where there is none; to stays to compress into form the swelling chaos of flesh; and to paints to rectify the dingy complexion. But in vain are all these attempts. No, if dissipation, late hours and immoderation have once wrecked the fair vessel of female charms it is not in the power of Esculapius himself to right the shattered bark and make it ride the sea in gallant trim again.

Thus spoke the famous beauty more than a century ago, yet her words are quite contemporary. Our skin does reflect the life we live and the food we take into our bodies. While no intelligent modern adult eats proportionately to the "ladies" described by Lola Montez, there is nevertheless a tendency to deny the body its proper rest and nutrition. We "burn our candles at both its ends," and we have been instructed from Biblical days to "take ease, eat, drink, and be merry . . . for tomorrow we may die." It is the rare individual who eats and drinks that which the body needs and conserves his energy with proper rest. Through the centuries we have seen fads in diet come and go with the changing modes of body beauty. I personally do not believe there is any set rule for food intake which is universal. I believe that the doctor who sets about to insist upon a rigid diet for his patient is in a class with Macaulay's bad government which would tell a man "what to eat and drink."

Each individual has different needs, and what might be a substantial food intake for one person could be a starvation diet for another. The one harmful factor of the on-again-off-again diet formula of so many people, insofar as the effect upon the skin, is the burden placed upon the elasticity of the skin and the forcing of an unnatural resilience. When one is quite young, weight can be gained and lost without much apparent damage. But as age encroaches, the diets which take considerable flesh off often age the individual more than aid—although the slender figure is naturally more youthful in appearance than the corpulent or obese. Your body and your skin require a well-rounded diet, and if you do not obtain the ingredients necessary in your food intake you should, under medical supervision, be provided with vitamin supplements to offset the deficiency created by the current fad diet. Contrary to popular belief, many diets make you look older rather than younger even though your figure is slimmer and your weight reduced. By denying yourself food you become nervous, irritable, subject to headaches and sleeplessness—and the result shows on the skin of your face.

If you wish to lose weight by dietary means, you should have a complete physical examination and then proceed to diet under your physician's care. In this way your skin does not have to be visibly affected and your aging process can be controlled by diet, in conjunction with proper exercise to avoid flabbiness.

That we live in a youth-oriented culture no one will deny, and no one can deny the importance of a youthful appearance in a day when the young people scream, "Don't trust anyone over thirty!" For years man has gone in search of eternal youth. The fountain of Ponce de León is a testimony to the quest, as are the many recorded diets, cosmetic ventures, and words of advice from both medical and lay writers. The search is varied and not entirely rewarding, but never ceases to invoke interest. In recent years, we have seen the advance of the science of gerontology—a branch of geriatrics in which man has attempted to take advantage of modern scientific advances not only to increase his longevity but to prolong his youth. There are many names which should be recorded among the youth doctors—some honorable and some fraudulent. Much of the experimenting among the youth seekers has been performed by non-medical people working outside the realm of accepted medical and scientific practices.

In the search for youth-restoring drugs, the American Food and Drug Administration (FDA) has adopted an ultraconservative policy. Sometimes it is many years before a new drug, used in animal experiments by the gerontologists, is released to physicians for use. Some European countries have a much more liberal policy and a new anti-aging drug is put into use as soon as it is proven safe for human beings. As a consequence, many affluent Americans take extended European vacations to visit one of the youth-restoring clinics. One of the most famous European youth doctors is Dr. Ana Anslan of the Parhon Institute in Bucharest, Rumania, who uses procaine injections to combat aging. Procaine (known also as novacaine) was discovered in 1905 by a German scientist, Dr. Alfred Einhorn. He used it as a substitute for the anesthetic, cocaine. In 1956, Dr. Anslan announced that over a seven-year period she had perfected a buffered procaine solution which could slow down and even reverse the aging process. Dr. Anslan called her mixture "H3" and it is marketed under the name "Gerovital." The treatment is given through deep-muscular injections administered three times a week. After twelve injections there is a lapse of two to three months and then the series of shots is repeated. Procaine injections have been used in Western countries since the late 1950s but the reports of success are conflicting. Because the injections cause discomfort and inconvenience, a German physician, Dr. Fritz Weidemann, in association with the pharmaceutical house of Schwarzhaupt K. G. of Cologne, refined a procaine drug which can be taken orally. The drug is known as "K.H.3 Geriatricum-Schwarzhaupt" or KH3. It is not marketed in the United States but is brought back to America by travelling Europeans. The Anslan and KH3 youth-restoring formulas are not based upon any particular theory of aging. The records kept by Dr. Anslan are not thoroughly scientific and Dr. Anslan has been openly hostile toward the criticism of the American Medical Association regarding her procaine treatment. She feels that many people are being denied the use of her formula because of our rigid restrictions. But to date the Anslan procaine method is not endorsed by medical authorities although a large number of prominent Americans have used the Anslan and KH3 treatment and profess satisfactory results.

Another European physician, Dr. Paul Neihans, is noted for his Swiss youth sanitarium. Many famous people have visited his clinic and claimed fantastic results. Individuals like Pope Pius XII, Bernard Baruch, Somerset Maugham, Charles de Gaulle and Gloria Swanson have sought renewed youth with Dr. Neihans.

Dr. Neihans' youth theory is one of "cellular therapy." He says he does not rejuvenate ". . . I revitalize." His treatment consists of injecting humans with living cells taken from the organ of fresh animal fetuses—usually lambs. The organs are cut into minute pieces with special instruments and are placed into a syringe and injected into the human. The fetal animal cells are supposed to replace something which age destroys in the human cells. The theory of cellular therapy has had a vogue in Europe—especially in Germany—but it has never been accepted by American and English physicians.

Aging actually commences when we cease growing and ceases when we die. In 1941, Dr. Johan Bjorksten established the theory of *cross-linkage* of materials in the cell nucleus as the principal cause of skin aging. Most random cross-linking—the process where the molecules that make up our cells and form the connective tissue that holds our cells together become cross-linked with other molecules—is harmless since the various enzymes in the body can break them apart. However, a certain percentage are chemically connected in a manner which prevents natural body enzymes from splitting them, and the cross-linking molecules can no longer function normally.* Your body contains many chem-

* Protein molecules contain sulfhydril linkages. When a rearrangement of the molecules occurs, there is a change in the physical pattern of the protein.

icals which cause molecular cross-linking, literally creating biological handcuffs. Some of the results are seen in the off-blance metabolism which occurs when more food is consumed than can be utilized by the body. This helps account for the fact that thin people tend to live longer than obese people. Excessive use of tobacco and alcohol, and exposure to noxious gases, can cause an accumulation of cross-linking agents which produce body and skin deterioration.

Cross-linking is not so important during childhood and adolescence when the body is growing and the cells are dividing. Then the cross-linking agents are evenly distributed between the new cells and the connective tissue between cells. It is when you have ceased growing and the cross-linked material in your body continues to expand that trouble commences. It begins to occupy more and more space in your body tissues and the gradual process of aging starts.

At the date of this writing, there is no valid scientific solution to the problem of cross-linkage. Dr. Bjorksten, under the sponsorship of the Upjohn Laboratories, is working on a theory, removing enzymes from soil bacteria which might break down cross-linked protein and thereby lengthen the aging process. Comparatively little research has been done on skin aging. To date scientists *do not* fully understand all the reasons for aging in the connective tissues of the skin or elsewhere in the body. We know that the aging of connective tissue cells plays a large part in skin aging, but it is probably not as essential as the biochemical reactions which take place. *Collagen,* the most important of all of the fibrous connective tissue proteins, plays a significant role in current research.

Collagen constitutes between thirty and forty percent of all the protein in the body and the total quantity of collagen increases with age. Furthermore, the collagen fibres themselves undergo radical changes during the life span. A thick matting of collagen forms the corium, which gives the skin its toughness and plasticity. The corium is the layer in the hide of animals which becomes the substance of leather after tanning and it is not insignificant that we refer to aging skin as "old and leathery."

As you have probably observed, your skin tends to age more in the epidermis of the face and the neck than elsewhere on your body. In 1961 the ultravoilet rays of the sun were pinpointed as the archvillain by Dr. John Knox, a fellow intern at Charity Hospital and presently Head of Dermatology at Baylor University. He has said that the onset of skin aging is independent of age, being determined simply by the cumulative amount of injury from ultraviolet light. The visible cutaneous changes usually interpreted as aging are apparently due largely, if not entirely, to sunlight.

The substantiation of Dr. Knox's claim lies in the fact that while your face and neck may be old and leathery your buttocks are youthful and firm. Those areas of the body which receive the least exposure to the sun and other external elements show the least ravages of time. But, as I have pointed out, one must not overlook the racial and hereditary factors, recognizing that Northern Europeans tend to be more prone to early skin-aging than those people whose ancestors came from tropical climates and whose pigmentation is darker, as those of Oriental stock.

It is not very practical in this day of sports and sports enthusiasts who are sun worshippers to issue an "out of the sun" ultimatum. Nor is it actually advisable or expedient, because a certain amount of physical exercise is essential to the toning and good health of the skin. With the problems your skin encounters in today's environment, then, what can your dermatologist offer as aid, beyond medical help for sick skin and general skin care?

RHYTIDECTOMY—FACE LIFT

The face lift is a surgical procedure performed by a plastic or cosmetic surgeon in a hospital. Its purpose is to remove bulges of skin and smooth out wrinkles. This is an extremely delicate procedure in which your doctor cuts through layers of skin behind the ears, above the hairline, close to the lashes of the eyes or in a natural skin fold of the neck-chin area. The skin is then stretched tight beyond the incision line and the surgeon sutures the incisions so the stretched skin will remain firm. The sutures are in place for a variable period of time. There are three dangers involved in the operation: 1) Some nerves may inadvertently be cut giving a partial paralysis to portions of the face. 2) There may be excessive keloidal scarring of the incision wounds. 3) The skin may be stretched too tight, resulting in a *frozen* expression which makes it impossible for the patient to smile normally. A friend of mine sent me a patient who had experienced such a face lift. She was a very wealthy woman who had followed fashion vogue and had undergone plastic surgery to lift her face. She was a jolly, outgoing woman who had a rather amusing raucous laugh and had a tendency to enjoy being "one of the boys"—so to speak—laughing loudly at the jokes of her men companions and contributing some rather salty ones of her own selection. The face lift had unfortunately frozen her wide grin, incapacitating her ability to laugh. The damage was irreparable—not only to her face, but to her spirit. Overnight she had become another personality, one extremely wearing on her own nerves. Under this stress she aged much more prominently than she would have in the natural course of time. Face lifting today by competent plastic surgeons is usually safe and accomplishes the desired effect—especially for professional people whose livelihood is dependent upon a continued expression of youth. It is an expensive procedure—the cost ranges from $5,000 to $10,000—and the results cannot be guaranteed. Comparatively few surgeons have mastered this very delicate technique. The face lift lasts from five to ten years and the body will not tolerate more than three such operations in a lifetime.

Under no circumstances should face surgery be undertaken by anyone other than the most highly skilled and competent cosmetic surgeon. Beware of bargains—and butchers. While your friend who recommends such a person may survive—you might not!

DERMABRASION

Dermabrasion or skin planing was one of the first cosmetic procedures to be perfected by dermatologists to cope with scarring. It is a much less severe procedure than face lifting and is done in your doctor's office. It can be limited to a small area of the skin and is used very often by dermatologists to remove the ravages of extreme acne.

The dermabrasion procedure is performed by the doctor after the skin to be planed has been cleansed as for surgery. The skin in the area is then frozen (usually with dichlorotetra fluorethane). This acts both to immobilize the skin and to locally anesthetize it, reducing the temperature of the skin below the point where the nerve ends conduct pain signals. The first dermabrasions were actually performed with sandpaper to remove the epidermis and the uppermost layer of the dermis. Later a small rotating wire brush was introduced. Today a small wheel or pear-shaped instrument, its periphery covered with diamond dust, connected to a high velocity dental-type drill, is used to gently scrape away the scarred area or that portion of the skin which shows signs of aging. Considerable skill is required to *feather*—or blend—the planed areas so that the line of demarcation is minimized. The danger in dermabrasion is a physician, who, lacking proper skill and dexterity, planes too deeply into the dermis and leaves permanent scars or produces changes in pigmentation.

The rotating wire brush ruptures the small blood vessels in the dermal skin layer and a certain amount of bleeding occurs during the planing. During the healing period (about two weeks) collagen and elastin molecules form in the uppermost dermal layer, replacing the cross-linked molecules planed away. A new skin, deriving from the deep pockets of epidermis in the hair follicles which have not been touched by the planing procedure, replaces the old. Like the skin of a newborn infant, it must be carefully cared for. This means very gradual exposure to the sun and other environmental factors which cause cross-linking of the molecules and the aging process of facial skin. Properly done, dermabrasion can produce very satisfactory results. It is most effective in removing pitted scars and excrescences (growths) produced by various skin diseases.

The cost of the dermabrasion is in the neighborhood of

$500.00 and upwards, and the time of inconvenience and reclusion is about two weeks. Again it cannot be emphasized too strongly—*know your doctor, and know his work before proceeding.*

CHEMICAL EXFOLIATION—CHEMOSURGERY

Chemosurgery or "dermalift" is more commonly known as the "face"—or the "deep" peel. The primary difference between the face lift or dermabrasion and *chemexfoliation* is the use of chemicals rather than scalpels or abrasives. It is a refined form of cosmetic surgery and now that it is an accepted medical procedure, it has certain advantages over the other two forms of surgery. 1) It is less expensive and less time consuming and painful than face lifting by surgery. 2) While the face lift rearranges facial tissues there is no change in the dermal and epidermal layers of the skin, whereas in chemosurgery there is a partial regeneration of the two skin layers and the connective tissues. 3) As a consequence the face treated by chemosurgery can be treated many times while the face lifted by surgery is limited in the number of operations that can be performed. 4) The cost of dermabrasion and chemosurgery range from $1,500 to $1,500 in contrast to the cost of the face lift by plastic surgery which ranges from $1,500 upwards.

It has on its negative side the fact that it was popularized in America by lay operators with little or no training in medicine. There were many incidents of scarring in the thirties and forties. When this occurred the patients sought the help of dermatologists and for a long time doctors shied away thinking it was too risky a procedure for practical purposes. In California, where the sun and outdoor life are especially damaging to the skin and where many of the residents are affiliated with the movie industry and its youth culture, all forms of face lifts came into their own.

The chemical exfoliation procedure became popular. The name Cora Galenti is associated with the early days of chemosurgery. Cora Galenti was a skilled operator—an artist who learned her techniques through some family connections who had earlier been in the business of facial rejuvenation. I have personally seen some of her successful jobs and have been impressed, but she had little or no knowledge of medicine and eventually ran afoul of the law and was forced to leave the country. Unfortunately there still exist lay operators who perform chemosurgery, and we doctors often see the results of their bad scarring and burning. For the most part doctors have improved chemical exfoliation and it is as safe as any of the other procedures and very often more satisfactory.

Interestingly enough the "deep peel" is probably the oldest known process for making the aging skin appear younger. Cleopatra was reputedly a skilled practitioner in the art of *peeling,* using the technique on herself and also on the ladies of her court. Her knowledge was inherited from the Egyptian physicians who had lived and studied medicine for a thousand years before Caesar and Marc Anthony. It was a young physician, Ptolemy, who first observed that when extreme sunburn caused the skin to peel, the new fresh skin appeared younger than the old epidermal skin that had peeled away. In performing peels, Ptolemy used the bark of oak trees which contained tannic acid and is not too unlike the phenol used in modern chemosurgery. Through the years the treatment was refined and by the time Cleopatra used it, it had reached a highly developed stage. The deep peel became a lost art after Cleopatra. Its secret was buried in the tomb of Ptolemy and the Egyptian Queen.

The light peel, using pumice and acetic acid, had already spread from Egypt to Arabia, and after Rome's conquest of Egypt, it reached European shores. Vanishing along with other medical knowledge during the Dark Ages, it began to reappear during the Renaissance, and by the time Marie Antoinette made her appearance, it was a common practice among the ladies in the court at Versailles.

During the nineteenth century, with the studies of Dr. Joseph Lister, phenol became a popular medical disinfectant, and about 1890 the deep peel appeared again among ladies and gentlemen of fashion. Unfortunately it did not reach the physician's office and become a part of medical care until recently.

The procedure of chemical exfoliation begins the day you decide you wish to wipe away the ravages of sun and age. It is most essential that you consult your doctor and tell him of the cause of your distress and the psychological motives in your desire to change your appearance. Because the after-care requires considerable self-discipline, your doctor will want to be assured that you are emotionally stable and that your decision is not a momentary whim. You should have a physical checkup before undergoing chemosurgery, not because it is a dangerous or traumatic experience, but because it is expedient to know your general state of health when undertaking a treatment which is going to tax your patience and test your ability to follow instructions to the letter for optimum results.

Some dermatologists and some patients prefer hospitalization, but a great deal of chemosurgery is performed today in the doctor's office and the patient assumes the responsibility for after-care. A male patient is clean shaven and a female has all cosmetics completely removed before the chemosurgery.

Liquid phenol (carbolic acid), trichloracetic acid or resorcin mixtures have been prepared in advance. Phenol is both an acid and an alcohol. Controlled caustic destruction by precipitation of the proteins of the superficial skin is the key to chemosurgery. If tissue is destroyed properly it will stimulate the body to regenerate new tissue. (Incidentally, there are no secret ancient formulas used in chemosurgery, and Cleopatra's secret has not been guarded by any one person and transmitted through the ages to a chosen few—a claim often made by "quacks.") A few minutes after the phenol is applied the skin turns white. Obviously, the patient has been given a sedative in order not to feel the stinging pain, and all efforts are made for comfort during the twenty to thirty minutes the application treatment requires. After the phenol is applied the patient is sometimes taped, sometimes not. The tissue destruction is instantaneous, regeneration begins immediately, and the next thirty hours is when the most important development takes place. The new elastin collagen and reticulin molecules will be more youthful and more pliable as in infancy and again will not be subject to cross-linking damage for many years. During the recuperative period, the patient is advised to abstain from talking and remain in as quiet a position as possible. Fluid intake should be in copious amounts (no alcohol is permitted) during the first few days. After a due period the skin forms a mask which dries and begins to peel. The peeling is done by your dermatologist. In the first stage the skin is very red and exposure to sunlight is not advisable. Under normal conditions at the end of two weeks the skin is regenerated and the red coloring begins to diminish. The annoying "crow's feet" have disappeared and although the skin looks younger and fresher there is not the unnatural look that many face lifts produce.

For at least ninety days following the treatment you have to avoid the sun and you should limit your intake of alcoholic beverages or stop them entirely. Vitamin intake should be ordered by your doctor and your diet should be a slenderizing one so that your entire being assumes the youthful appearance of your face.

The changes in your face depend upon your subjective reaction to the treatment you have undergone. Miracles do not occur in the office of your doctor any more than they occur in some form of psychic phenomona. Certain results can be produced by plastic surgery, dermabrasion, chemosurgery, but the end result of any form of beauty aid you undertake must be in the image you have created within yourself. The result you see in the mirror will reflect the image you wish created for yourself. If your dermatologist could play a Pygmalion role and create the physical image you desire, could he also play the psychological role and alter your identity? Shaw could accomplish the change in Eliza Doolittle's appearance but it was the telltale words of Professor Higgins that gave substance to the true love interest with his wistful words, "I've grown accustomed to her face. . ." Of all the aids we can summon—and I believe we should summon all we need—we must also recognize that neither the surgeon's knife, nor the dermatologist's formulas, can recreate the essential human visage.

HAIR AND NAILS

"We have been, let us say, to hear the latest Pole,
Transmit the Preludes, through his hair and finger-tips."
—T. S. Eliot, "Portrait of a Lady"

As we noted, the appendages of your skin are indeed a part of the bag you live in and an integral part of the skin itself, though these are often regarded as things apart.

Next to the "skin you love to touch," the human hair has a more decided effect upon your interrelations with other human beings than any other external feature. People react strongly to the color of one's hair, its kinky, curly, or straight appearance, its texture and odor.

Dandruff, for example, is a common scourge which has been deplored for centuries. Oily hair, which requires almost daily washing, is a trial and a tribulation to those who possess it. According to fashion, the curly or uncurly tendencies of one's hair is of vast importance. The question of hair color has reached such proportions of commercial absurdity as to generate the "Do blondes have more fun?" and "Does she or doesn't she?" questions. And we who live once again in the age of wigs have become acutely aware of the importance of hair to the individual's vanity. Hair transplants—both expensive and tedious to execute—are performed daily not only on celebrities but on business men and society matrons to preserve the illusion of youth which supposedly diminishes with balding hair or an early loss of color. Shakespeare said, "Her hair shall be whatever color it please God to make it." This was true in the sixteenth century, but modern cosmetics have made fallacies of such truths. Hair has become the easiest of all the skin's manifestations to alter; but in the altering one must expect to pay certain prices. More money is spent annually on cosmetics for the hair than for *all* medical research in this country. With proper knowledge you can care for your hair correctly and make it a crowning glory for inner good health and beauty. The state of your health is sometimes evidenced in the condition of your hair.

Phylogenetically, the hair or fur—that most characteristic feature of all mammalian skin, including human—serves mainly as a protection from exposure and for attraction of the same species. The plumage of the male bird is used in his courtship of the female to attract her attention. In the case of some animals, the porcupine for example, the quill which replaced the hair or fur acts as a passive defense against attack.

In the human the hair has diminished in extent by evolution. Its thermoregulatory protective function been replaced by the wearing of clothes, although hair follicles continue to be found over the entire body of man, with the exception of the palms, soles, surfaces between the digits, and a few other very limited areas. Hair in and around the openings of the nose, ears, and eyes, moreover, helps to protect against the admission of harmful particles or stray insects, as the hair of the scalp provides a cushion for the head while aiding in insulation. In areas such as the groins and armpits, hairs act as roller bearings, protecting two adjacent skin surfaces from rubbing irritation. Although the function of the hair in thermoregulation of the body temperature has been preempted, the ancient mechanism of involuntary contraction of the tiny *arrectores pilorum* muscles, attached to the base of the individual hair shafts, are still demonstrable when you become chilled or frightened and develop "goose flesh" or "goose pimples." Your hair rather literally "stands on end." Hair generally occurs only sparsely on the limbs and trunks of females (although there is a wide range of *normal* hairiness, or hirsutism), being confined largely to the pubic area, the armpit and the scalp. Except for plucking, shaving, or the use of chemical or physical depilatories—all of which are temporary measures—the most effective current method for the permanent removal of unwanted hair is by electrolysis. This is tedious, painful and expensive, but, in the long run and in the hands of a good operator, effective. In the male, hair distribution is greater than on the body of the female. Thick hair growth occurs on the pubes, armpits and scalp, in addition to the bearded area of the face. In humans, the downy hair of the fetus is replaced in the eighth or ninth month of pregnancy or in the newborn period. The pubic and axillary hairs appear in adolescence in association with the development of secondary sex characteristics at puberty. Some loss of scalp hair generally occurs in the large majority of males after pubescence, in early manhood, particularly at the frontal margin of the forehead. This results in a somewhat *M*-shaped hairline. Again, during the period of senescence in both males and females, there is a more generally diffuse loss of hair in the scalp, armpits, and pubes, coinciding with that period of life during which the sexual powers and appetites are supposed to diminish—the climacteric, or change of life. Throughout all this period there is a steady coarsening or thickening of the calibers of the individual hairs over the entire body, and, frequently, a loss or modification of color, either darkening or lightening. Many people believe that hair growth in the male is somehow associated with potency and virility, thus the prevalence of hair transplants among celebrities whose popularity depends to some extent on their image of sexuality and virility.* The hairy man is generally supposed to be more powerful physically and more potent sexually than his nonhirsute counterpart. He is more readily identified with the primitive man, the uninhibited, sexually aggressive, violent, pre-historic male who cornered his mate as she came around a boulder in the Stone Age, socked her on the head with a club and dragged her off to his cave to enjoy the massive forces of his sexual powers. Contrary to this, observers as early as Aristotle note that eunuchs do not bald; it has been firmly established that a normal complement of male hormones is necessary for the develop-

* One of the few exceptions to male virility being associated with the non-balding male was the performance of Yul Brynner in *The King and I* in which Mr. Brynner portrayed the King of Siam with a bald pate. His sexuality was so apparent that there was a vogue of association of sexual prowess with the totally bald man. The illusion was largely Mr. Brynner's.

ment of the common pattern of baldness in men. Baldness can also occur pathologically in some women whose hormonal make-up has been radically altered, for example, by the presence of masculinizing glandular tumors. Methods of wearing the hair vary in both male and female from society to society. Today long hair is in vogue for both men and women. Just a few years ago long hair on a man indicated effeminacy, while short hair on a woman implied masculine tendencies. In ancient Crete both men and women removed all hairs from the body, and men wore their scalp hair at the shoulder length of today's male hippie. In Renaissance Europe and Elizabethan England, wigs flourished—in England perhaps because of the early baldness of Queen Elizabeth and Mary, Queen of Scots—among both men and women. In the early days of our country long hair was favored among both men and women. It was not until the day of the flapper—just after World War I—that the short hair style for women became acceptable, let alone popular. Coco Chanel originated the style and Zelda Fitzgerald, through her husband Scott's writings, immortalized it in *This Side of Paradise* and *The Great Gatsby*. Aldous Huxley also wrote of "bobbed hair" in the year 1933:

> The longer our fathers thought, the better. How the heart beat, as the loosened bun uncoiled its component tresses! And if the tresses fell below the waist, what admiration, what a rush of concupiscence! In many, in perhaps in most, young men at the present time long hair inspires a certain repugnance. It is felt vaguely, to be rather unhygienic, somehow a bit squalid. Long hair

has become the non-conductor of desire; no more does it attract the lightning. Men's amorous reflections are now otherwise conditioned.

In addition, D. H. Lawrence, author and advocator of female emancipation and sexual freedom "bobs" the hair of his Gudren and other heroines as a symbol of thc changes in western civilization and the invasion of women into fields formerly identified solely with men.

But, to many women and to many men, long hair is a "thing of beauty and a joy forever." The Scripture tells us "if a woman have long hair, it is a glory to her."

There are a great many primitive rituals and customs involving cutting and dressing of the hair. In many of these an aggressive component may be discerned, as in the custom of some tribes of the American Indian of scalping one's enemy and then proudly displaying such trophies. Certainly the Biblical story of Samson and Delilah is an inherited tale of castration through the shearing of Samson's locks by Delilah, thus depleting him of his source of exceptional strength. It is definitely of some significance that we constantly say we will not "harm a hair of his head" especially in view of the fact that hair, itself, is totally insensitive. This common human vow, reiterated through the ages, seems to spring from some deeper interpretation, some form of folklore handed down through the ages and never dismissed.

The hair on one's head is totally removed in our society under certain circumstances. For example, formerly it was shaved in monks and nuns who had disavowed the sexual life and chosen the celibate. In some areas it is shaven off convicts, not only, one may assume, for the practical purposes of identification and hygiene, but also as a part of the penalty society imposes upon its enemies—symbolic scalping. This scalping is used when women in occupied countries collaborated with the enemy through sexual intercourse with the soldiery. In the world of Synanon, where drug addicts have attempted to cure one another and live together without the use of drugs, a bald head is a sign that the shaved individual has slipped and again used drugs—the haircut is an outward sign of his backsliding and is administered by the group as a form of therapy. The shaving of one's head is often used as a means of protest, as was recently witnessed when the young girl-followers of Charles Manson appeared with their long, flowing tresses shorn to the scalp in protest against society's judgment against their leader. Often shaving of the head is used by doctors as a means of eradicating a bothersome skin disease of the scalp. In military societies, for the most part, the short crewcut is useful for the early detection of vermin and for cleanliness. In some countries and in some circles, hair length is determined by compulsory regulations. Only recently has the United States Navy relaxed its restrictions on hair length for enlisted men and draftees.

Hair growth in man is cyclical. There are various stages of early formation, resting, and sloughing off, followed by a repetition of this cycle. The length of the cycle and its components varies in different hair follicles and particularly in different regions of the head (longest on the scalp, where the cycle in some women may last several years).

The human hair grows fastest on the scalp and chin areas. Hair grows faster on women than on men. On the average individual hair grows approximately five to six inches per year. Hair grows faster by day than by night (due undoubtedly to the increased metabolism during the waking hours). Hair also grows more rapidly in hot humid climates and faster during the summer months. Between the ages of fifteen and thirty, hair grows most excessively. Hair commences to thin, bald, or grow more slowly from the age of forty-five.

Unlike other animals, there is not a simultaneous wave of growth and resting in the hair follicles of man; consequently, he does not molt. The facility of growth seems to be inherent in the hair follicle itself, and depends little on outside influences. For example, contrary to popular belief, shaving does not increase the rate of growth or change the texture of the hair shaft. After shaving, there seems to be a temporary increase in the growth rate followed by a compensatory slowing of the rate, amounting ultimately to *no* change. Also, the hair does not grow after death, as is commonly supposed. The skin about the hair follicles merely recedes, giving the mistaken impression of growth.

Hair is a symbol of human emotion when man attacks his own hair and pulls it out or attacks and pulls out the hair of another. The emotions involved are grief and rage. In grief, man often destroys his own hair and in anger he reaches for the hair of another. (This latter exhibition is more commonly associated with women in their fights.)

The hair of man falls and is replaced cyclically from birth to death, and when the old hair fails to be replaced by new, thinning known as *alopecia* results. One particular type of this condition is *alopecia prematura,* or hereditary male baldness. Another is *alopecia areata,* or spot balding, seen in both men and women and occurring in the scalp, beard, eyebrows, lashes, or wherever there is hair. (Women, by the adjusting of their coiffures, can often more carefully conceal alopecia of the scalp than men, and for many years were not publicly known to suffer from this disease.) Spotty baldness is of unknown origin, although emotional duress is often noted, and hormonal factors may play a role. The condition may spread to involve all the hair of the body; it is then known as *alopecia universalis,* and even the nails may be affected. Treatment with some of the cortisone and cortisone-stimulating preparations has been effective. One important condition which will mimic this type of spotty baldness is another patchy but moth-eaten looking loss of hair caused by syphilis. Other more exotic diseases will cause a similar appearance, but the most common cause is the *alopecia areata.* This is neither infectious nor communicable, and frequently responds well to treatment. Psychosomatic factors are very important in the etiology of this condition. One often finds a predisposition to neurosis among sufferers. The factors generally considered to cause childhood insecurity, such as parental disharmony, divorce, separation, alcoholism, and poverty, are usually also apparent in the studies of alopecia. Thus, a rigid family structure, either patriarchial or matriarchal, or a situation in which all forms of self-assertion and self-aggression are unacceptable, can result in a head covered with only patches of hair. A small child once described a male guest who suffered from the disease as the "man with the holes in his head."

A survey of the personality patterns of sufferers from alopecia indicated that the most striking feature of the male patients in the group was their lack of drive. This permeated their whole personality, affecting their social relations, work, sexuality and aggression. There was a general tendency to avoid competition and responsibility. Although many patients studied had never received what they considered their just deserts in life, they accepted their failure with characteristic apathy and resignation. Many of the men in the group expressed overt fears of sexual activity and they rarely achieved satisfaction in sex relationships. All of the male patients associated sexuality and alopecia. The single men were markedly inhibited in the realm of sex; masturbation was infrequent and feared as weakening and harmful; many had preserved their virginity beyond the usual age and some only indulged in homosexual relationships of the most infrequent and heavily guilt-ridden nature.

The women patients in the same group were sexually immature. Their heterosexual relationships were boy-girl platonic friendships. Among the married patients there were many who had achieved a father-daughter relationship, seeking to be their husband's little girl. Full sexual happiness was not common and many marriages had failed because of the patient's lack of response.

Naturally among women the loss of hair was more frightening than among men. The single girls believed their chances of marrying had faded and those who were married feared their husbands would seek another mate. All of which indicates that women also associated their alopecia with a diminution in their powers of sexual attractiveness.

All of the patients were predisposed to psychological instability and the neurotic symptoms had preceded their alopecia. The alopecia added to their burdens and aggravated their anxiety or depressive symptoms and reinforced their underlying emotional insecurities. There is little evidence of the coincidence of psychoneurosis and alopecia, but the occurrence of alopecia is closely related to a psychoneurotic condition.

There are many instances of a patient relating how his baldness developed "overnight," frequently following intense shock, and in many cases the precipitant being a situation which caused acute fear or anxiety; many of the cases are related to soldiers in action. One very famous actor whose child was victimized in a kidnap told me his hair turned grey and began to "fall out" at that moment. In this group the personality patterns are quite diverse. The threats of danger have very often been directed against some individual other than themselves, but all of the victims stress the fact that the shock is something totally unexpected. The physical symptoms which preceded the hair change were feelings of acute anxiety with trembling, palpitation, feeling faint or as though the head was going to burst, and a tingling up the spine and over the occipital part of the scalp. There is no permanent psychiatric disability in these cases and a reasonably successful adjustment to the situation which caused the alopecia can bring about the regrowth of hair.

In addition to fear, the impact of grief can create external evidence in the loss of hair. In *Mourning and Melancholia* Freud takes the view that the death of a love object requires that all love attachment *(libido)* be withdrawn from the object which no longer exists. This withdrawal requires a struggle since man never willingly abandons a love attachment. The process of detachment is carried out over a period of time, bit by bit, and when completed the mourning ceases. In *Melancholia* Freud suggests that the lost object is incorporated into the self and consequently feelings of love and hate originally directed toward the other person become self-directed. On this basis he describes the loss of self-esteem and self-depreciation which characterize melancholia. Since pulling of hair is associated with the emotions of fear, anger and grief, it can be assumed that instances of alopecia phenomenologically constitute a concommitment of pathological grief or fear, and the loss of hair represents an unconscious attack against one's self.

There are many more tangible types of alopecia, some causing scarring and others not. Thermal, radiation, and caustic burns; bacterial, viral, and ringworm infections; tumors; and scarring skin diseases can cause scarring alopecia. High fever and toxic states, congenital defects, chemicals, hormones, skin disorders and psychopathological conditions can cause the nonscarring type. Pulling the hair too tightly in pony-tails or around curlers or the neurotic disposition to deliberately pull out one's own hair *(trichotillomania)* can occur. *Defluvium* (loss of hair) can occur following shock as readily as following excessive exposure to radiation or the ingestion of such drugs as thallium. Broken, falling hair is a feature both in ringworm of the scalp (which is virtually never seen in adults) and in chemical damage from the use of cold-wave solutions (thioglycollates) or hair straighteners (strong alkalies).

As we observe the adjectives relative to the feel and look of skin we note that the poet sings of the golden, soft, brown, silky locks. He speaks of hair, so "charmingly curled," "soft-lifted by the winnowing wind" and scented with the "mist of rain." Until recent years there was little mention in praise of the kinky heads of a considerable portion of the world's population. For many years, kinky hair was something of a curse and many men and women spent large amounts of money on the sundry processes of "hair straightening." Perhaps even more than the color of the black man's skin, his kinky hair—which he attempted to straighten with greasy pomades—alienated him from social contact with his white brother. In the South, where I was born, it was customary for many years that black customers be unable to try on hats in stores before purchasing. The hat to be bought was purchased ultimately on the basis of buyer's imagination or salesman's persuasion. This custom was the result of the heavy usage of grease which remained on the inside of the hat when it was removed and consequently made it undesirable for sale. The fact that a white customer using an excessive amount of brilliantine or "sta-comb" could induce the same results was overlooked and yet another form of discrimination was sustained. In the social evolution of the American black, the first sign of economic success was the abolishment of the kinky hair with which the black person was born. In the forties, fifties and sixties most successful blacks had their hair *straightened,* but again with the emergence of African power and an appreciation for cultural values today's black beauty wears kinky hair proudly as a symbol of freedom and equality. While most of the body hair has a tendency to curl, the hair on the scalp varies in accordance with its genetic origin. One inherits naturally curly or wavy hair, just as one inherits one's natural hair color and one's natural predisposition to a luxuriant growth of hair or an early predisposition to balding or greying. Most efforts to offset that with which one is born are artificial in stimulus and sometimes successful, sometimes injurious. Like the skin, your hair reacts to inner physical and mental health and the forces of environment. Like your skin, hair dries with overexposure to the sun and heat rays, and like your skin, it dries without a supply of essential body oils.

Scalp stimulus—such as brushing or massage—is of minimal importance in the maintenance of a healthy head of hair. Cleanliness is most essential, whether by brushing or washing; an excessive accumulation of the unsaturated fats from the sebaceous glands and other detritus will eventually lead to some falling out of the hair. There are those who keep their hair clean and luxuriant with little more than moderate brushing with a natural-bristle brush; others—generally with a more oily scalp—require frequent shampooing. Unless scalp disease is present, a mild shampoo, *e.g.* castile, is usually adequate. Over-washing without adequately removing the soap or detergent particles can produce a dry, itchy scalp, however, and the ensuing scratching can cause loss of hair. Dyeing, which was once hazardous, is today reasonably safe—provided you do not possess an allergy to the ingredients in the dye, or you do not use a product which destroys the hair in the process of changing its color. Body-hair dyeing is more hazardous than scalp-hair dyeing and most manufacturers of dye products warn you against the use of dyes on the eyebrows, eyelashes, body and genital hairs.

HAIR TRANSPLANTS

Most dermatologists are aware of the vital role hair plays in the human life, since hair is a part of the organ we specialize in. But even we are not fully conscious, at times, of the impact of hair on human behavior and what men and women *will* and *do* pay to have or not have hair.

It is estimated that $500 million will be spent this year just for wigs and hairpieces, and the sum allotted to hair care in men's and women's beauty parlors and hair styling salons is about $7 million—exclusive of the sums spent in doctor's offices to offset some of the damages created both by nature and by man himself in his quest for—hair!

In the past decade the offices of dermatologists have been filled with both men and women seeking relief from balding, itching scalps. The mental anguish of these patients is very real and often devastating.

Your dermatologist has worked at cures for the skin diseases of the hair mentioned in this book, but the results are not phenomenal. However, one of the more recently developed treatments can be performed successfully and with little discomfort for the patient—that is, the hair transplant for baldness.

If you wish a hair transplant, consult your dermatologist who will explain the procedure to you. In most cases, the operation is performed in the doctor's office with the use of a local anesthesia.

Your doctor draws the desired hairline in gentian violet. If you have advanced pattern baldness, your doctor will do a receding hairline rather than one close to the original. Once the new hairline has been agreed upon, the donor area starting with the occipital region of the posterior scalp, is clipped with scissors to outline an area of about one by three or four inches.

Both donor and recipient areas are then anesthesized with

2 percent xylocaine and epinephrin. The most satisfactory punch sizes appear to be 4.5 millimeter for the donor plugs and 4 millimeter for the recipient holes. The two different punches make a much better fit of graft to transplant site and apparently better healing and less scar formation.

Grafts are taken in two or three rows, with fifteen to twenty in a row. Normally twenty to twenty-five punches are needed just to outline the new hairline.

To cover the front hairline of a male seeking a hair transplant would require sixty or more punches. The cost of the punches would range from $10 to $25 per punch depending upon the individual doctor. The hair transplant is an extremely expensive procedure especially if a large area of the head has to be replanted.

It is important in the transplantation to make certain that the grafts are placed so the hair grows in the proper direction. They should grow anteriorally in the anterior part of the scalp and toward the back in the posterior region.

Once the grafts have been inserted, both the donor and recipient sites are checked for bleeding and once dry, they are covered with Telfa dressings with an antibiotic ointment. Dressings are left in place overnight and you are advised to sleep in a semi-sitting position and avoid rapid walking, stooping over and vigorous chewing. To minimize the possibility of edema, a one week course in corticosteroid therapy in diminishing doses is occasionally given.

The day after the grafts, the bandages are removed and the hair properly washed in your doctor's office. Frequently, you are then advised to start daily washing of the scalp in the shower, using plain water. Often the hair in the donor plugs will fall out, but new hair will begin to appear in about three months and in time your baldness should be ameliorated, although naturally the hair is never quite as thick as it originally was.

With strict adherence to this routine I have yet to see a transplant fail to offer beneficial results.

The results are usually very satisfying to the patient, producing in both men and women renewed physical vigor and interest in life. The fact that many prominent individuals have had transplants—one of the more famous being the transplant of Frank Sinatra—has made them popular and less cumbersome than expensive wigs and all of the sundry remedial lotions and usually unrewarding preparations bought and sold over the drug counter.

In regard to transplants the real question is—how much does your hair mean to you? If it's worth the price of a transplant which runs approximately $10 to $25 per 4 millimeter plug, then consult your dermatologist and proceed.

EXCESSIVE HAIR

Since the beginning of time women have tried to get rid of superfluous hairs using various methods, but most depilatory measures do not give a permanent result; rather they produce a heavier and coarser growth of superfluous hair and some manufactured diplatories are disastrous for use by those individuals who are allergic to their contents.

The plucking of heavy brows has been an accepted custom for years. You can usually do this in a satisfactory manner yourself with a pair of eyebrow tweezers. Application of a vaseline compound to the skin before plucking makes the procedure easier and applications of witch hazel following the act diminishes the redness and temporary swelling. The hairs should be pulled out one at a time and the pain can be eliminated by pressing the skin near the hair, pulling the follicle down from the hair shaft.

The razor and pumice stone can be used to cut off hair and smooth the skin but as the hair grows again, shaving has to be repeated more and more often and the young hirsute girl commencing this form of hair removal in adolescence can be shaving as frequently as her boyfriend.

Depilatory creams, pastes and resins are available, but the hair returns very shortly after their use. The active ingredients of these products is sulphate of barium, or strontium. It is spread on the skin and allowed to harden. When it is removed it takes away the offending hairs. In order to avoid an eventual dermatitis from this procedure, wash and neutralize your skin with some acid solution, lemon juice or white vinegar, and then smear or dust the skin with a soothing cream or powder. The skin looks very good after the treatment with a dipilatory but the hair returns very shortly and again after several applications it coarsens and becomes more of a nuisance.

Application of hydrogen peroxide in a solution 10 to 15 percent can often be effective in the bleaching of a dark hair hirsutism. The solution should be combined with 2 or 3 percent ammonia. The best method of application is to apply cotton at the end of a stick, soak the cotton in the mixture, and soak the hairs until they become colorless. The ammonia dissolves the fat of the hair making it easier for the hydrogen peroxide to get to the hair and bleach the melanin. After the treatment, the skin should be covered with a cream to soothe the area. In the bleaching of body hairs, the peroxide affects the horny layers, causing them to break, which is advantageous on the body; but the same form of hair-lightener when applied to the scalp has a deleterious effect. Since the hair grows rapidly and the new hair or roots will again be dark, the procedure has to be repeated quite often.

Unusually heavy development of human hair is called *hypertrichosis.* Those suffering from this condition are as miserable in their plight as those individuals who are afflicted with baldness. Hypertrichosis in men is important if it makes them appear ape-like. More important is hypertrichosis in women.

Excessive hairiness starts during puberty when hair in girls begins to appear in regions other than those characteristic of the female sex. Hairs of moustache and beard appear and the genital hairs extend upward to the navel and heavy hairs grow around the nipples of the breast and between the breasts until they join the abdominal hairs. They also appear in abundance on the thighs and on the forearms, chiefly on the extensor sides. In short, your female body commences to resemble the hairy body of the male.

Hypertrichosis is a disease sometimes but not always connected with the internal secretory glands—especially the sexual glands. In some cases, it causes the young girl to develop a masculine personality and often the hairy appearance creates a Lesbian personality in the growing girl.

Hypertrichosis increases with advancing age, and because of the masculine identification many young girls become embittered. Supersensitivity about their disease develops a mania and sometimes they even commit suicide. Many threaten the latter, and to offset an increasing neurosis when their physical condition interrupts romance or interferes with their normal sex life, it is most important that the condition be remedied as soon as possible. When the treatment is successful it is most gratifying for your dermatologist to see the visible change in personality and witness a *joie de vivre* replace a sullen depression.

The role of your dermatologist in cases of hypertrichosis is important—for if the case is severe you eventually will have to consult a dermatologist for hair removal. There are several methods employed. One is epilation by X-ray. This method is obsolete and extremely dangerous if applied injudiciously or with the wrong technique. When done in a wrong manner you can be subject to Röntgen burns which sometimes (even years later) can result in ulcers or keratoses which ultimately will become cancerous.

A drug, thallium, can cause epilation when given orally. It is a highly dangerous drug and was formerly administered only to children with ringworm of the scalp. It is no longer a part of the dermatologist's armamentarium.

The best methods for extirpating the body hairs permanently are found in *electrolysis,* where each hair papilla is destroyed with an electric current or by a high-frequency current—*diathermy.*

Electrolytical epilation must be performed by an experienced electrologist. In the hands of a skilled operator it is an efficient but painful and time-consuming method for the permanent removal of superfluous hair. It can cause tiny, scarcely visible scars in some cases but, when well performed, the rate of regrowth is negligible. It is an operation done without anesthesia. One of the most important features is a proper prognosis on the part of your doctor in which he tells you following an examination just what results may be expected. It is extremely difficult to foretell the length of time necessary for electrical epilation of a very hairy region or a thick beard. The correct estimation of the number of hairs to be removed is a difficult task and only possible after great practice. It is nearly always several times greater than the patient thinks. The operator generally uses one or two types of machines—either a *mikrostat* or a *pantostat.* With a needle he probes the follicle and finds the papilla of the growing hair and destroys it by the current of electricity. The quickness and success of epilation depends very much on the patience of the patient and the skill of the operator. The few hairs which do regrow will appear shortly after epilation but the extirpation of these few hairs is quite easy. For example, if a few months were required to remove a heavy face beard with daily sittings of half an hour each, the after treatment would only require one or two sittings a month—the sittings lasting from a quarter to half an hour. The principal disadvantage of electrolysis is that even with the best equipment and the most skilled operator, the procedure is a very tedious one and therefore should be used only for facial hairs.

For excessive body hairs, removal by *diathermy* is more practical.

Diathermy is the transformation of electrolytes of high frequency currents into heat. It is the most perfect method of heat application because the heat does not pass in from outside by conduction or radiation but a high frequency current conveyed into the interior of the body causes heat to be produced in the cells themselves.

NAILS

The nails, those hard, keratinous appendages which form at the ends of the fingers and the toes, are important areas of the skin. The fingernails with which we indulge in scratching are especially important. "To scratch the part of the body that itches" is the height of human happiness, according to Thomas Carlyle.

Your fingernails are the leading agents of disaster to the rest of your skin. They are the prime carriers of skin infection and the army of busy, surgically sharp instruments which dig unmercifully into the skin upon your conscious or subconscious desire. Most of the filth that penetrates beneath the surface skin reaches its destination by means of the dirt which accumulates under the fingernail and is transmitted through the innocent, pleasurable scratch to other skin areas. The fingernails deploy or destroy the natural contour and beauty of the hand, and their care has become an industry within the cosmetic industry—the manicurist and pedicurist being specialists in their field.

The nails portray to the trained eye the racial genetic source of the owner, even though upon occasion the rest of the skin denies the heritage, and the nails are telltale beacons of many physical ailments which have not yet disturbed from within. Today, the use of fingernail polish has become so commonplace that it is almost unique not to see a woman with painted nails—yet, not so long ago such painting was a trademark of the working whore. Today the lady sits with, "Each fingernail a crimson petal seen Through a pale garnishing of nicotine." (Robert Hillyer) Except in the case of bitten nails, carelessly attended nails or overly exaggerated long nails, the individual trying to analyze the owner by fingernails would not dare to draw some conclusions which once existed. For example, in the history of witchcraft and werewolvery, the length of the nail and its habit of turning under were considered outward evidences of the demon existing within. Today when long, slender, highly polished nails are the epitome of fashion, and the envy of persons who do not possess them, one would hardly dare to summon past allusions. Yet certain men cringe at the sight of long fingernails, associating them with tools of torture if the owner becomes angered and starts to fight and scratch with her natural-born shears.

Tickling, itching and diffuse burning pain all represent the same sensory quality and are felt in turn as the intensity of a stimulation is gradually increased. The urge to punish oneself or to exorcise the evil can be expressed in the form of scratching and erotic needs may be gratified by stroking or rubbing one's self. Naturally, the condition of the nail is most essential in any of these acts.

Deformities and disfigurations of the nails can happen from a variety of causes: a complete congenital absence of the nail plate; a crushing physical injury of the nail root resulting in ridging, reeding, fluting, or a marked thickening of the plate; weakness, degeneration, and detachment of the nail from its bed by the excessive use of "frosted" nail polishes or commercial household detergents or, paradoxically, the application of "nail hardeners." Because some three months or so is required for the normal fingernail to grow out, and about six months for the toenail, and because of the relative inaccessability of the components of the nail to treatment, therapy is often distressingly long and drawn out.

Other conditions affect the cuticles and tissues about the nails—hang nails, ingrown nails, warts, moles, tumors, fungus infections. In addition, many nail disorders are seen in association with and manifcstations of other diseases, either internal or external, and should be approached with that consideration in mind.

DISEASES OF THE SKIN

As you now know, skin diseases are manifold. Those listed and detailed in this section are the more prevalent, therefore more easily recognized by the lay reader.

Some of the tragically serious skin ailments such as *pemphigus* (a continuing formation of large blisters on otherwise seemingly normal skin) are rare and, therefore, primarily of academic significance. They have been by-passed in this section of the book which is intended primarily for lay-reader consumption. These diseases are of serious prognosis and are sometimes fatal. Requirement for their medical care is imminent and the diagnosis is customarily followed with the need for immediate professional attention.

To the healthy, all disease is a bore, a scourge. The healthy individual might find the following chapter on skin diseases boring. The hypochondriac, on the other hand, finds disease thrilling and relishes the subject. He is inclined to indulge in reader identification and in the chapter on skin diseases he might find a sort of smorgasbord or juicy skin orgy.

But the prime purpose of these words on certain skin diseases is to give you some helpful indications of a skin ailment so you might recognize the symptoms and receive proper medical care before the disease has passed beyond the nuisance stage; and to alleviate unnecessary fears regarding skin eruptions and disfigurements and to offer simple remedies and precautions.

Essentially it is important if you are concerned with the condition of your skin that you consult a trained doctor; if you are imagining skin fantasies perhaps you will be able to relieve your mind and worries by easily acquired knowledge of common skin diseases—the symptoms and the available cures.

If you wish to by-pass the reading of sundry skin diseases and are only concerned with your particular skin ailment or problem, the diseases discussed are listed alphabetically below for your convenience, reference and research.

> There is no such thing as a purely psychic illness or a purely physical one, but only a living event taking place in a living organism which is itself alive only by virtue of the fact that in it psyche and soma are united in a unity.
>
> —Francis Mohr, M.D.

It is amazing how far medicine has been able to progress on the basis of the conception of the human organism as being essentially inanimate—rashes, masses, breaks, the filling up of orifices and the depletion of vital supplies. When we have thought about it as being in action we have thought in terms of a machine with a good or bad motor (the heart), and some doctors and institutional researchers have in the past chosen to study it in a form as free from actual daily living as possible—in the *basal* state of the bed.

This has all changed and today's doctor is trying to understand the human organism as one which responds to stress of all forms—from deprivation of essential vitamins to deprivation of human affection; from the compensatory overdrive required by a *mitral stenosis* to that created by a sibling rivalry.

With this concept of modern medicine, your skin has taken on a new and more exalted role. Not only does your skin stand between your inner and outer world, but the great interplay of forces is reflected in its functioning. Today your skin is not only a means of insulating, weatherproofing, cushioning and covering you, but it is also a barometer which sometimes reveals inner illnesses or tensions, and indicates a state of systemic disease not otherwise apprehensible.

The study of medicine has passed through a morbid descriptive era in which changes observed in the organs and tissues of those suffering or dying were written about and recorded accurately for centuries, to the present day when the greatest attention is being given to the normal and abnormal ways in which a man reacts to his surroundings. In short, medicine has travelled from a study of anatomy and histopathology to physiology and psychology. Disease may appear to affect only an organ or a part of an organ, a tissue or a system, but a disorder in any part of the body must to a lesser or greater degree affect the whole being and reflect some disturbance.

Skin is your largest organ, it is also your largest area for expression of internal ills. You are an individual personality; with your own attitude of mind and your own way of reacting to life; you are not just a cancer, asthma, or dermatitis case history.

Two generations ago your family doctor knew you from the moment of birth until the moment of death (if not he, his son who traditionally inherited his practice). He knew your background, the conditions of your conception and birth, the problems of your personal environment, your tolerances and intolerances, and he had some understanding of you and your personal problems. But it was not until Sigmund Freud and those who followed him that study of psycho-dynamics became of scientific value. In a very brief description: this approach was an attempt to place the understanding, friendly doctor-patient relationship on a scientific basis. The method involved a careful simultaneous study and treatment of psychological and somatic factors in their organic interplay. It became referred to as *psychosomatic medicine.* Such a title has been ridiculed and has often been misinterpreted in parts of the medical and the lay world. Unfortunately, we live in a world of labelling and this particular label has been damaging, but its truth is almost perfectly exemplified in the study of you and your skin.

Granted some skin diseases are local reactions to outwardly acquired infections, physical or chemical injuries, but many are manifestations of the presence of internal organic diseases, including emotional stresses. For example, easy bruising—"I bruise if you touch me"—is a warning signal to look further for the possibility of an existing blood abnormality or a vitamin deficiency, and constant scratching until a skin abrasion causes you to come to a dermatologist for a relieving salve may be the outward manifestation of a deep inner emotional disturbance which has been so repressed and controlled that in the process of self preservation the skin finally has let forth the howl which the mind could not or would not allow the human voice machine to utter.

You also may consult your dermatologist with a skin ailment which you in your modern medical sophistication attribute to "nervousness"; you blame your work, your sex life, your social existence as being the cause of your "nervousness" while you refuse to accept the fact that your skin may be a canvas upon which is clearly painted for your doctor to see—a personality defect. Jean Charcot, the famous neurologist, developed at Salpétrière in Paris the greatest clinic of its time for nervous diseases. Among his patients was the Marquis de Sade. Charcot's pupil, Freud, credits him with being the first to isolate hysteria as a psychological problem. It was the great Charcot who said, "We see only what we are ready to see. We eliminate and ignore anything that is not a part of our prejudices."

Historicity plays a most important part in the study of skin diseases and therefore an honest and well-reflected open history is probably as important in the diagnosis of your skin problems as in the other, unseen areas of medicine. The use of various laboratory techniques, including the examination of a small, superficial plug of skin under the microscope—the common biopsy—can tell your doctor much, but a true history of noxious contacts—animate, physical or chemical—such as bad diet, drug taking, emotional stress will fill in the gaps and give your doctor the chance to connect the effect with the laboratory tests much more accurately than if he merely diagnoses your condition from the laboratory slides before him.

No disease is static. It is an active, ever-changing process of adjustment which affects your whole personality, bodily and mentally.

You must learn to live with unfavorable inborn traits, racial and family influences, types of upbringings, acquisition of bad behavior patterns, occupational and social customs which you accept or against which you rebel, for it is a combination of adjustment to all of these factors, in addition to many other purely physiological factors, which establishes your state of health. Your skin is an outward manifestation of your adjustment.

As Alexander Pope wrote, "The proper study of Mankind is Man." The most perfect study of you is you and the skin which reflects you. As early in the history of man as the writings of Plato we find the admonition to those doctors who had dismissed the Hippocratic outlook and committed "the greatest error of our day . . . the physician who separates the soul from the body . . ." And Shakespeare's Lady Macbeth, guilt-ridden to the degree of madness, cries out, as she rubs her murdering hands: "Out, damned spot . . . out!" Whether or not there were actual spots is, of course, controvertible, with inscrutable guilt being the prevailing force. It is quite possible, however, that she could have been afflicted with one of the psychologically related dermatoses: hives, perhaps, or a less common one, *erythema multiforme,* which also can be precipitated by extraordinary emotional stress. The latter is a disease where bright red spots appear, generally on the extremities. It seems to have a connection with the allergies, and is one condition which, in addition to others such as hives, migraine, and asthma, can be instigated by intense and heavily bridled mental distress. America's own Louis Adolphus Duhring first isolated the disease and wrote a treatise on the subject many years after the tortured Lady Macbeth had wandered across a stage haunting many and audience-filled theatre with her pathetic cry "Out . . . out. . . !"

The cause of many skin diseases remains obscure to this very day. They are variable in characteristics and are subtle in their gradations from one type of reaction to another. In this day of sundry types of external chemicals—solvents, detergents, lubricants, the reaction of one skin may differ from that of another. For example, several years ago, one of the leading cosmetic firms brought out a new fingernail polish. It contained an ingredient which was disastrous to certain nails, while harmless to others. The effect on a significant number of nails, however, was enough to recall the product and the firm was obliged to pay heavily for those incidents of serious physical damage resulting from its usage. There are many basic reasons for skin disturbances, among them:

1) Your inherited racial and genetic qualities and faults which will cause individually different types of skin reactions.

2) Your skin has to withstand all sorts of physical conditions—climatic, seasonal, occupational, extremes of heat and cold, humidity and dryness, and has to adapt itself to knocks, rubbings, scratching throughout the night and day.

3) As we live in an age of synthetic chemistry, today your skin is exposed to an ever-increasing number of chemicals which can be harmful. In short, one man's nylon may be another man's poison.

4) Parasitic, viral, and bacterial causes. Although

there are perhaps fewer parasitic diseases than there were a century ago, there nevertheless does exist a sufficient number of skin diseases due to such origins that it is a noteworthy source. A person who develops a rash, for example, after exposure to his favorite cat, and learns that his skin is in a constant state of irritation because he fondles his pet, is always alarmed that the irritating cat fur or the parasite which might be thriving on the body and in the hair of his beloved pet is the source of his personal skin ailment. He is then confronted with a dilemma which can create an emotional disturbance as well as a physical one. Such cases are seen daily by every practicing dermatologist. Recently a very proper lady came to me with a very disturbing skin malady. Much to her horror and my embarrassing discovery, she was the victim of bites from "bed-bugs." In view of the fact that she lived in an upper-class neighborhood and she associated such a problem with filth and poverty, conveying the truth was not a simple matter. Fortunately, it turned out the luxury apartment she rented was a sub-let and she was not responsible for the condition. Even so, she was mortified to learn that her mysterious rash was a scourge of parasitic origin—the lowly, but devastating "bed-bug." *Scabies,* caused by the itch mite, is a particular nuisance in our mobile society, particularly in colder climes and in the winter months with the wearing of heavy clothing. Head and body lice continue to breed. The eyelashes of one infant patient who had been travelling with her parents in the Near East were completely covered with the parasites, and had to be treated with the regular application of yellow oxide of mercury eye ointment and the manual removal of the individual nits from the lashes with forceps.

Diseases caused by viruses include *herpes simplex* (cold sores or fever blisters), *herpes zoster* (shingles), and various types of warts.

Among the bacterial diseases is impetigo—highly contagious in infants and children—which can sometimes become ulcerative, after which it is known as *ecthyma.* There is *erysipelas* and *erysipeloid* – commonly seen in butchers and fishermen—carbuncles and furuncles, and infections about the hair follicles and cuticles. Tuberculosis of the skin and leprosy can appear in different forms, and fungous infections can either be of the superficial or deep variety.

5) Nutritional deficiences have a hypersensitive reaction on the skin. Beware of bad diets or faulty methods of preparing your food in order to avoid a form of *avitaminosis,* advanced forms of which can show up as beriberi, scurvy, or pellagra.

6) Diseases which reach the skin through the blood or lymphatic streams—frequently eruptive disorders such as *syphilids, tuberculids,* and *dermatophytids.*

7) The influence of endocrine glands on your skin.

8) Degenerative changes of the skin, whether from aging or other circumstances.

9) Emotional stresses which play some part in the inception, aggravation or maintenance of dermatosis, or alone can be responsible for abnormal skin aberrations.

"My skin is broken and has become loathesome," moaned Job of Biblical lore. It is true that skin diseases are usually thought of by the lay mind as nasty, dirty and infectious. A patient of mine who developed an environmental allergy to mites confessed to me that she thought she was being "punished" because she had always been the owner of "the skin you love to touch" and had been repelled all of her life by unattractive skin. When her own skin underwent a physical change, she underwent simultaneously a complete psychological change. Her normal extroverted personality went "underground"; she withdrew from society at large and confined herself like a recluse, or a "leper" (as she once described herself). Her style of clothing—she possessed a beautiful figure—changed, and she refused to wear anything that did not cover the mutilations her skin had suffered.

Itching has been associated with parasitic infections such as the itch mite or the louse. Today itching is more often caused by some central or peripheral stimulation of an overexcitable neurocutaneous apparatus.

With few exceptions skin diseases are not lethal. Consequently they seem less important and less dramatic than diseases affecting vital internal organs. They are associated with unpleasant crusting, scaling and ulceration and may be abhorred because of fear of contagion. This fear persists although contagious skin diseases are located in very few patients today.

Many skin patients and their friends and relatives regard skin diseases as being due to dirt, and think that those who suffer from skin diseases should be avoided like the plague. This is the reason for the mental condition termed the "leper complex."

A person with extreme dermatosis may meet with great difficulties throughout life. In childhood there is often cruel ostracism and ridicule. It is often impossible for a skin sufferer to join in sports such as swimming or to be eligible for such recreational facilities as summer camps. In later life holding down a job can become something of a problem due to complaints of fellow workers. Marriage may be deferred or avoided because of a skin malady, or after marriage, friction and disharmony over one's mate's bad skin can even result in divorce. It is not uncommon for victims of skin diseases to feel themselves outcasts from society. The penalty is especially cruel in view of the genetic history of many skin diseases.

With the exception of eye diseases and skin deformities, which can evoke sympathy, skin diseases are the only visible maladies of mankind. The repugnance is probably related to the fact that the decomposition and decay of the tissues is identified with death. You can suffer from a peptic ulcer, cirrhosis of the liver, or brain tumor and you will be allotted a large degree of sympathy because of the drama associated with these ailments and the fact that they cannot be seen by the naked eye—but skin disorders are obvious, ugly and only too often not understood in matters of origin and lack of contagion.

The emotional effects of a skin disorder vary enormously from one individual to another. There are many people whose skin disorders occupy their minds to the exclusion of all other matters. It depends to a great extent upon the vanity of the individual. A blemish on the skin can very often be a peg upon which to hang innate fears of cancer and other diseases.

The origin of the word "blemish" is not certain. It is defined as a physical or moral defect, and consequently, the smallest skin lesion can alter your entire personality, if it concerns your feelings about your physical or moral welfare.

You must be aware that your skin can be definitely affected by the state of your mind, either directly or indirectly. For example—

1) The symptoms or signs may be wholly psychogenic.

2) The emotional factor is more important in your reactions of hypersensitivity.

3) A normal emotional manifestation in your skin may be maintained unduly by your mental attitude toward your condition.

4) Emotion may be one of the causes for setting off or aggravating skin viruses.

5) Emotional disturbances may predispose you to skin infections.

6) Emotional conflicts may lead to over-exposure to venereal diseases; or increase the chance of drug intoxication or the risk of dermatitis by the excessive use of soaps or antiseptics; or expose you to malnutrition through dietetic fad.

7) The gratification of itching, if inhibited in one skin area, may be satisfied in another because one area is forbidden.

8) A vicious circle of mind-body-body-mind aggravation can occur, as in *acne vulgaris.*

9) Emotional disturbances can seriously affect and create occupational dermatitis.

You may work for years exposed to skin hazards but remain unaffected until some emotional conflict causes you to "break out" and become allergic to your work and place of work, thereby necessitating a radical change. Often when a skin disturbance due to working environment occurs, anxiety ensues and fear of losing the job intensifies and irritates the condition further. In addition to the anxiety there also occurs a resentment that you are affected by the environment while your co-workers remain unmolested. The result can often be such a radical personality change, followed by unemployment.

10) Persons with strong masochistic and exhibitionistic tendencies often exhibit a perverse need to appeal for sympathy with some form of self-disfigurement. It is frequently, but not necessarily, seen in those with a consuming phobia to the "creepy-crawlies," and such victims will attack themselves ferociously with weapons ranging from cuticle scissors to caustic soda, inflicting unsightly scars in their tightly secluded orgies of self-mutilation, while steadfastly denying their morbid acts even in the face of overwhelming evidence to the contrary. This type of ailment is highly resistant to cure, and even when checked, often reappears for no explicable reason, in spite of psychiatric treatment from eminently qualified practitioners.

11) Trivial, small or mild lesions in your skin may cause such mental distress that the condition is aggravated and often resistant to cure. For example, *alopecia,* which is associated in the mind with sterility or impotence, can get completely beyond control as a result of the accompanying anxiety.

In relation to all diseases of the skin you must first remember that the skin you are born with is inherited and largely influenced by genes. With a history of parental skin ailments you can be on the alert and take the proper care and caution and help preserve your skin in the best possible condition. Knowledge, removal of false superstitions and beliefs of contagion, acceptance and adjustment, and proper medical and personal care are the key words to better skin health.

As we have noted, the number of diseases of the skin exceeds a thousand, so we will concern ourselves only with the most commonplace—those you are most apt to encounter in yourself or in acquaintances.

12) The manifestations of skin diseases are divided into two groups—subjective and objective. The former, called symptoms, are those endured by the patient alone as a result of his personal sensations and observations. The other, called signs, are those seen by the naked eye or detected by a physician in his investigation of the disease. Some diseases of the skin have associated symptoms in which the cutaneous lesions are merely one expression of the general pathologic process. The importance of an accurate case history in relation to all skin diseases, so the doctor can properly diagnose the disease, cannot be overemphasized.

Chief among the symptoms of a skin disease which you might suspect are sensations you can observe beyond the visual—itching, burning, smarting, prickling and tingling. Other sensations are apparent when your skin comes in contact with foreign bodies, sensations of increased or diminished temperature; pain in various grades of severity; feelings of the crawling of insects (even though nothing is apparent to the eye); and compressions of portions of your skin as if tightened by a rubber band or a cord. You are conscious of all of these sensations before they become evident to another eye, or even under a microscope. They are your own built-in detection devices.

The importance of the study of objective signs cannot be overemphasized since it is with a clear understanding of these symptoms that your doctor can make a proper diagnosis.

The signs of skin diseases are called *lesions* and it is customary for doctors to describe them as *primary* and *secondary,* or *elementary* and *consecutive.*

In discussing primary lesions doctors and patients communicate by using ordinary objects to indicate size. You tell your doctor you feel a lesion the size of a pea, a poppy seed, a chestnut, the egg of a hen or the commonplace pinhead.

The next important word for you to know in relation to skin diseases is *macule,* which is a circumscribed alteration in the coloring of the skin of varying size and shape. Macules may be congenital or acquired and may be the only cutaneous sign present or may represent an actual skin eruption. They may be some shade of red, yellow, brown, or occasionally, white. They may be due to pigmentation as in the case of freckles, or they may be associated with the escape of the coloring matter of your blood into the skin area. Macules also may be injected into the skin with dyes such as in tattooing, or the explosion of gun powder near the surface of the skin. Extensive skin color changes occur in some systemic conditions such as yellow fever, cancer, Addison's disease, and metal poisoning. These are not macules.

Papules are circumscribed solid elevations of the skin, varying in skin size and round or irregular at the base. The top may be pointed, acuminate, conical, rounded, flat, or depressed in the center. In color they may be bright red or dark red or deep brown or dead white. They may be located anatomically around the hair follicles or any portion of the skin's surface. They may be transitory or persistent. They may be scaly or a pustule may develop on their surface. They may produce a sort of colony of growths or they may be transferred into other lesions of the skin—being self-infectious. They may have the sensation of feeling or they may be devoid of all sensation.

Pomphi are circumscribed, more-or-less transitory, elevations of your skin, ranging in size from a pin-head to the size of your hand. They are accompanied by itching, tingling or prickling sensations and usually appear and disappear rapidly. They are usually red in color and occur following insect bites, or food allergy or rash. They are referred to as "wheals."

Nodules are rather persistent, solid elevations of your skin, varying in size from a pea to a cherry. They range in color and are different from papules in size. They may be individual or grouped and they frequently develop into ulcers and occur characteristically in syphilis, leprosy, sarcoma and carcinoma.

Tumors are new growths of varying size and composed of any of the structures of the skin or subcutaneous structure. They may be solid or compressible, benign or malignant. They may be located within or beneath the skin and may be attached to the latter but project from it a variable distance. In size they vary from a walnut to enormous growth of great weight. They are not common in most skin diseases but are seen in fibroma, sarcoma and carcinoma.

Vesicules are circumscribed elevations of your skin containing fluid. They may be individual or grouped and may be transitory or of long duration. They frequently dry and become crust-covered. Sometimes they are itchy and sometimes they are not.

Pustules are elevations of the skin ranging in size from a small seed to a filbert. They can assume many shapes and can be superficial or deeply rooted. They contain pus, and when the fluid becomes encrusted, it causes the crust or scab to assume the color of the fluid. Pustules are seen in syphilis, scabies, acne, and many forms of dermatitis.

Bullae, or blisters larger than vesicles, are superficial or deep-seated elevations of the skin containing fluid. They range in size from a pea to a goose egg or even larger. They change in size and color and, like pustules, contain a lymph or fluid. They may be thick, or thin and easily ruptured. They may dry and form crusts or they may become ulcerous. They are classically seen in leprosy, erisipelas, syphilis, gangrene and common burns and scalds.

Secondary lesions are dried areas usually resulting from imperfect cornification.

Scales. Scaling is a prominent feature of many skin diseases. Scales may be fine, brawny, dirty white, yellowish or pearly white and shiny. They may be dry or fatty, few or abundant, firmly or loosely attached. They may be aggravated so as to resemble a pie crust or exfoliate in extensive sheets from the palm of the hand or the sole of the foot. They may fall in quantity on the bed sheets or on the patient's clothing causing embarrassment and an appearance of physical messiness.

Crusts are composed of dried serum, pus, blood or extraneous matter. At times they are comparable to dried honey, gum or tree turpentine. They can be delicate and thin, or bulky and thick. Sometimes they separate easily from the skin and sometimes they are almost inextricable. They range in size and color and are especially commonplace in impetigo, eczema, leprosy and syphilis and many other minor diseases of the skin.

Excoriations are usually the result of excessive itching and are most commonly produced by the fingernails. They are seen in all of the itchy diseases of the skin and in time a skin long-scratched will become thickened and pigmented.

Fissures occur as a rule in a skin which has lost its elasticity through infiltration and thickening. They occur most commonly where the extensibility of the skin is essential to accomplish the necessary movements of the parts—the hands and feet, finger ends, palms and soles. They are frequently painful and interfere with walking and use of the hands. They often occur with the aging process of your skin.

Ulcers differ greatly in shape, size, color, edges, base and history. Every ulcer has an outline, a base, a floor, edges and secretion. Ulcers may or may not be crusted and they may or may not be painful. They may heal or remain open indefinitely. They appear in syphilis, carcinoma and leprosy and they often occur in the lower extremities as the result of secondary infection caused by congestion due to varicose veins. They can occur from bedsores in cases of general debility. Ulcers terminate after healing with cicatrization (the forcing of the formation of scar tissue).

Scars are new formations of new tissue replacing tissue lost through a destructive process. Scars may be minute or cover vast areas. Sweat pores and ducts of sebaceous glands and hairs are absent in scars. Subjective sensations rarely accompany scars, though some are associated with itching and minor pain. In early stages they are red and later become pigmented or remain white. Scars may result from any injury to the skin or any form of skin disease which involves the loss of the connective tissue elements of the corium.

So much for the technical physiological evidences of the hundreds of diseases to the skin. They may range in seriousness from a casual sunburn blister to a blister indicating a profound malady. Only a professional eye can discern the difference. Many eruptions of the skin are infectious but very few are contagious. Even the virulent spirochete of syphilis requires some break in the integrity of the skin—some fissure, howsoever minute—to gain a portal of entry into, and a means of infecting, another body.

Leprosy, for example, requires very prolonged and intimate contact for transmission and, even so, many racial types offer pronounced resistance. In Carville, Louisiana, where the only leprosarium in the continental United States is located, there has been no incident of leprosy being contracted from patient to attendant in the more than a century-old colony. In studying skin diseases, and in attempting to understand skin conditions to make life more pleasant for yourself and your neighbor who may suffer from a skin ailment, it is most essential that you remember—at all times—that the most infectious skin disease is *self-infecting* but not, of necessity, contagious. Most of the contagious skin diseases are the childhood epidemic diseases such as chicken-pox, measles, impetigo and certain venereal diseases. These latter are highly contagious because of the mucous areas of penetration which are easily vulnerable and therefore easily susceptible to contagion. Today these illnesses, which were thought to be on the decline, have increased in such abnormal proportions that the occurrences of venereal diseases are almost epidemic in size, and obstinate to the use of the sulfa drugs and antibiotics which a generation ago were considered "fool-proof."

Your skin presents frightening spectacles to you and to your social acquaintances, but in many instances your unattractive surface covering is only harmful in the irritation it is causing you and the interference it is creating in understanding between you and your neighbor. It is with such an outlook that I will brief you on some of the skin diseases which seem most formidable.

CANCER

Cancer is one of the greatest killers of mankind. In the United States it causes about 305,000 deaths a year—more than any other ailment except heart disease. Skin cancer, the most prevalent cancer, is the most curable form of the disease. About 85,000 people in the United States will develop skin cancer this year. Hopefully, most of these will use common sense, see their doctor early and be cured, since the cure rate is very high—90 percent. Most doctors believe if the skin cancer is apprehended in time, the present death rate would subside considerably.

Skin cancer, like all forms of the disease, is an uncontrollable growth of abnormal cells capable of invading adjacent tissues and organs and spreading throughout the body.

The normal growth of skin cells is when the cells divide to

replace worn-out cells, and repair injured tissue. Cancer cells grow in an unregulated manner, without constructive purpose. They choke out normal tissue as they spread to adjacent tissues. Cancer cells can also break away and spread to different parts of the body, a process called *metastasis.*

Because your skin is your largest organ and performs so many varied duties, it is constantly subject to injury by infectious or irritative agents. Resulting abnormalities which occur are usually benign. However, abnormalities can and do sometimes lead to cancer.

Certain abnormal-skin diseases which have a tendency to become cancerous are known. The most common is *senile* or *actinic* (sun-ray) *keratosis,* sometimes classified as "precancerous."

A keratosis is a small skin thickening which usually develops in an exposed part of the body such as the face or the hands. Senile or sun-ray keratosis usually develops in an older person whose skin has been exposed to the sunlight many years.

Cancer can and does develop in almost any area of the skin. The exposed parts—face, neck, forearms, and backs of the hands are the most common sites.

Skin cancer may appear as a dry scaly patch, or a pimple which persists or an inflamed area with a crusting center, or as a pale, waxy, pearly nodule which may eventually ulcerate.

Malignant *melanoma,* a relatively *uncommon* cancer of the skin, occurs usually as a dark brown or black mole-like growth which may increase in size rather rapidly, and, at times, may ulcerate and bleed. It can arise from a persisting "mole," although some melanomas do not. A patient of mine, for example, had a dark mole in the left corner of her chin. It was a family "mark" and seen in three generations of family portraits and referred to as the famous "Graham beauty spot." In the days when other ladies wore patches for beauty's sake, my patient's illustrious forebearers did not have to do so—nature had endowed them with the traditional mark of beauty. But when her mole began to grow and then to ulcerate and bleed, it was no longer a "thing of beauty and a joy forever." It was a malignant growth—a blemish to be extirpated by surgery. In study of the case histories of her ancestors, the telltale melanoma was also a forewarning of the presence of the malignancies which took their lives at very early ages. In her case the surgery and after-treatment resulted in a complete cure.

Only your doctor can determine the nature of an abnormal growth, whether it is benign, precancerous, or cancerous. *You should immediately bring any skin change to the attention of your doctor.* If you do not have a doctor, consult a dermatologist as soon as you perceive a radical change.

If the doctor thinks your skin condition may be cancerous, a bioposy is performed. This is where the whole lesion or a fragment of suspected tissue is removed surgically and examined under the microscope.

The two main forms of therapy for skin cancer are radiation therapy and surgery, the latter including chemosurgery and cryosurgery.* In some cases a combination of treatments may be used. One treatment may be sufficient, but at other times more treatments are required. Each lesion and each

* Formerly radium was used extensively in the treatment of skin cancer (as well as many other skin diseases), but it is rarely used by the modern dermatologist having been replaced by X-ray and some recently discovered and developed treatment modalities.

patient is considered individually by the physician in deciding which treatment will produce the best results medically and cosmetically.

The principal cause of skin cancer is the ultra-violet rays in the sunlight. I cannot overemphasize the danger of overexposure to the sun. Other less common causes are excessive exposure to coal tar, pitch, arsenic compounds, paraffin oil, radium and X-rays.

Anyone can develop skin cancer, but it occurs most often in people who have fair, ruddy, or sandy complexions and are exposed to sunlight in excessive degrees. For example, farmers or sailors are highly susceptible as well as outdoor workers who live and work in the sunny regions of the world. Contrary to many peoples' thoughts, black people are not immune to the dangers of the sun. Skin cancer is occasionally seen among the black field hands and day laborers.

The greatest preventative against skin cancer is—*stay out of the sun!* Certainly excessive exposure should be avoided at all times. Protective clothing such as sun hats, long sleeves and gloves should be worn by those exposed to the sun for long periods at a time. There are some oils and lotions which have already been mentioned, but their effectiveness is limited. Sunbathing (although high fashion magazines encourage seasons in the sun for beauty) is indeed very dangerous. It not only increases your risk of skin cancer at a very early age, but it has a marked effect in prematurely aging your skin, thereby making it more susceptible to skin cancer.

Every day medical science is doing more and more research into cause and cure of skin cancer. Doctors are constantly trying to learn more about the maturing process of the skin in order to understand what happens in the change from normal skin growth to cancerous skin growth, but the best medical advice I, or any doctor today, can give you in regard to skin cancer is a simple therapy which is complete in your control: avoid the sun's rays, and when in the sun protect your skin in every possible manner to prevent overexposure. Even if your friends make fun of you and tease you about your reluctance to sun-bathe, remember my words of advice and stand fast by the scientific truth concerning you and your skin. Let the other person parch and age and ultimately develop skin cancer—be less glamorous, but be glamorous for a longer period of time. In the long run, you will be the winner and your sun-worshipping pal, the loser.

PSORIASIS

Psoriasis is a disease we hear mentioned on TV and radio commercials and see references to in all of our publications—yet there is actually very little known about the disease which is one of the most annoying and most cosmetically disastrous of all of the skin disorders. The primary cause of psoriasis (probably a biochemical fault) is unknown. What is known is that psoriasis affects the mechanism which the skin has for the manufacture of new cells. In unaffected persons, skin is replaced every three to four weeks, but replacement takes only three to four days in psoriatic skin. This excess skin production accounts for the characteristic scales of psoriasis. Some recent studies support the theory that heredity plays an important part in psoriasis, but the events which "trigger" the onset of the disease are multitudinous: injury to the skin, streptococcal infection of the upper respiratory areas, emotional stress. Psoriasis tends to improve during the summer months and many patients find relief from their suffering by living in such geographical areas as the Virgin Islands where the temperature remains in the seventies year round and where the tradewinds keep the body temperature at an ideal level. The connection between the geographical locale of the Islands is also indicated by the fact that psoriasis is not too common a skin ailment among black people, especially those who do not leave their native environs for colder climates.

Psoriasis comes and goes at unpredictable intervals. It is a flaking skin eruption and appears as plaques of raised red skin covered with white scales. Most areas of the body can be affected, but psoriasis commonly involves the knees, elbows, trunk and scalp. Fortunately this skin affliction does not cause pain or intensive itching.

Regardless of the appearance of the patient suffering from psoriasis *there is no fear about getting the disease by contact* and if you are a victim *you need have no fear of transmitting it to another person under any set of circumstances.*

The most important factor in your psoriasis is *your mental attitude* and the attitudes of those people with whom you are intimate. There is no reason to fear psoriasis. It does not cause cancer, nor loss of hair, nor does it leave scar tissue. It is most cosmetically unpleasant, but it is not serious and it is not associated with serious medical complications. Having psoriasis does not mean you are unhealthy, and control of the disease is possible if you follow your doctor's orders. A significant number of patients experience prolonged periods of complete freedom from the disease, but unfortunately and more commonly, psoriasis usually accompanies the patient throughout life. The best remedy is to control the rash as well as possible and the program requires careful planning and regular supervision. You should definitely be under a physician's care if you suffer from psoriasis, for there is not a pill with which to cure the disease, nor any ointment. Your physicians will prescribe a topical application of ointments, creams and liquids containing corticosteroid hormones, tar, and salicylic acid.

The use of shampoos containing tar and salicylic acid, the application of surface medications with gentle but thorough rubbing, and careful removing of scales with a soft brush are all important. Sometimes ointments and creams containing corticosteroids work better under a thin plastic film such as Saran Wrap. This treatment is called "occlusion" and is usually used no more than twelve hours a day and no more than one-third of the body surface is covered at one time. Vitamin therapy and diet are apparently not effective with psoriasis patients but obese patients with the disease improve significantly when they lose weight. Psoriasis is one skin disease which responds to careful sun- or violet-ray treatment.

Psoriasis also responds to combined physical and psychiatric treatment. In the study of the disease we doctors have come to recognize that patients with psoriasis show personality deviations prior to the onset of the disease. The patients are *compulsive* types who pay meticulous attention to detail and work until in a state of utter exhaustion, *overagressive* types with an intense resentment of authority, *underaggressive* types who suffer from inferiority complexes and often develop psoriasis during or prior to a nervous breakdown, *phobic* types who have phobias of bugs, filth, etc., during early childhood—all can develop psoriasis. In sort, a study of a group of patients suffering from psoriasis will reveal personality defects from mild anxiety to hysteria. Consequently, the relieving of the pressure causing the personality illness often will relieve the physical apparition of the disease. One patient of mine was a man who inherited a very wealthy business which he disliked but felt obliged to carry on in the family tradition. In the course of his attempt he became obese, developed acute psoriasis and even a tendency toward alcoholism. He went through three disastrous marriages with women who married him for his money but could not adapt themselves sexually to his repulsive body. One day after consulting with a psychiatrist, he sold his family business and retired to the Virgin Islands. In time he went into a small business utilizing his former avocation and hobby as a vocation. In the warm climate, removed from the pressures he could not sustain, he began to recover. He lost weight and his psoriasis disappeared. In time he married an understanding, intelligent woman who was no part of his former existence. Except for few occasions (usually when he is obliged to return to New York and momentarily encounters the same frustrations and problems which upset him previously) he has little or no trouble with his "terrible psoriasis" and is as happy as most individuals can expect to be.

The social effect of psoriasis is considerable. The appearance of the disease conjures up thoughts of filth, venereal disease and neglect. The onlooker will often flee in repugnance or ask embarrassing questions. This only aggravates the patient's condition. After the first attack, the patient wonders if the disease will reappear. He questions his right to bring children into the world and pass his curse onto the third and fourth generation and his personality, even if normal at the onset, becomes badly mangled in the course of the disease. Few sufferers from psoriasis derive much satisfaction from the fact that it is considered a "healthy man's disease."

The isolation which is sometimes self-imposed, but more often imposed by one's fellow men, is little compensation. To the sufferer I would say, adjust to your psoriasis, mentally and physically, and try to bring a sane adjustment in the people with whom you come in contact. This, and proper medical treatment, is the solution to your always-temporary cure.

ECZEMA

Skin conditions loosely described as "eczema" comprise about one-third of the dermatologist's medical practice. They are often recurrent and occasionally chronic maladies and tend to be refractory to treatment. There are many theories as to their etiology, yet there are hardly any two authorities who will concur.

Eczema is decidedly a protean disease. It is not only protean in its clinical manifestations, but its causes are varied, numerous and usually complex. The term eczema implies a "boiling over of the skin." There are eight principal groups of eczema: 1) contact dermatitis; 2) allergic dermatatis from within (due to food, drugs—penicillin being an excellent example of a drug which produces an inflammatory skin condition in those individuals allergic to its use; 3) infantile dermatitis; 4) seborrheic dermatitis; 6) infectious and parasitic dermatitis; 7) metabolic dermatitis and 8) dermatid.

Contact irritants, both animate and inaminate, drug intolerance, foci of infection, nutritional and metabolic disorders play roles of varying importance, but the factor of emotional liability, so often found in association with eczema, must not be overlooked.

In 1930, John Stokes of Philadelphia published isolated cases in which the frictional dermatoses rose in a perverse attempt to satisfy a sexual urge. In 1932 he named the personality of asthma-eczema-hayfever patients as the "tension frame of mind" and later commented upon their tremendous drive, restlessness, and overambitiousness. The importance of feelings of security and inferiority, overdependence and narcissisim, latent aggressiveness and egocentricity are noted among sufferers from eczema.*

Eczema is characterized by heat, redness, itching or burning sensations, infiltration of the skin, weeping or moisture at some stage, and multiform lesions.

Redness varying in shade from the bright red of the acute

* Scott Fitzgerald's brilliant but erratic wife, Zelda, who was diagnosed as a schizophrenic, suffered from eczema. Fitzgerald, in *Tender Is the Night*, gives a description of her agony:

> On her admittance she had been exceptionally pretty—now she was a living agonizing sore. All blood tests had failed to give a positive reaction and the trouble was unsatisfactorily catalogued as nervous eczema. For two months she had lain under it, as imprisoned as in the Iron Maiden. She was coherent, even brilliant, within the limits of her special hallucinations.

Zelda's personality from childhood was typical of the eczema sufferer, as the reader of Nancy Milford's best-selling *Zelda* (1970) can attest.

to the dull red of the chronic forms is present in all cases. Itching is practically always present and may vary from slight annoyance to intolerable distress. It is commonly intermittent in character and is usually worse at night. Occasionally the skin is hypersensitive to even the blandest of substances and patients have been known to require satin sheets and pillow cases to alleviate itching while trying to sleep. The degree and character of the subjective skin sensations in eczema depend largely upon the location, type and severity of the disease and upon the general physical condition of the person and the psychological peculiarities.

"My emanation far within;
Weeps incessantly for my sin."
—William Blake, "A Divine Image"

The internal factors, inducing sensitization, are errors of metabolism. Schamberg and Raiziss found true nitrogen retention in patients suffering from eczema of internal origin and Schamberg and Brown found an excess of uric acid in the blood; Klauder and Brown found that the calcium and potassium ration in the skin affects its susceptibility to irritation: increase in calcium diminishes, while increase of potassium heightens this irritability. Certain foods appear to be associated with atopic eczema: milk, eggs, pork, tomatoes, strawberries, nuts, chocolate and sea foods. Also inhalants of dust, feathers and animal furs can create an eczema condition. In some instances hyperthyroidism has been identified with eczema, and the patient cured by proper thyroid injections.

A long list of diseases is commonly enumerated as being the cause of the patient's skin eczema, but the diseases are now believed to be only contributory factors. The diseases are: acute rheumatism, diabetes, nephritis, asthma, disorders of the liver, anemia, tuberculosis and syphilis. The victims of gout and rheumatism often do have a form of chronic eczema and the association of eczema and asthma is commonplace.

Nervous shock and prolonged mental depression are definitely important factors. In the treatment of children affected by eczema it is very often more important to treat the parent rather than the child patient, for affected children and adolescents seem to be overstimulated and overambitious and it is necessary to reduce internal conflicts to a minimum. When the atopic dermatitis continues on into adult life, one often encounters mother and father complexes which develop during childhood, and the treatment requires a psychiatrist in addition to a dermatologist. One patient at the Menninger Clinic, for example, had eczema which had penetrated her vaginal area. She attributed her problem to caring for her senile, diabetic father who also had incontinence. In her analysis by Karl Menninger, it was revealed that her real problem was her Lesbianism which had been present for many years and which she feared would become known in the community in which she lived.

There are many cases of hormonal imbalance in women with an abnormally dry skin. There are cases of premenstrual aggravation and a history of the skin condition clearing up during pregnancy or developing at menopause. However, it is generally conceded that this form of eczema is more closely related to hyperestrinism than to a deficiency of estrone.

Eczema may result from contact or occupational dermatitis but this usually occurs after prolonged exposure. Some of the susceptible vocations are: baker, confectioner, dyer, printer, tobacconist, grocer, ink manufacturer, painter, gardener, laundress—occupations which necessitate working with cement, chemicals, synthetic resins, cutting oils, etc.

In susceptible persons acute eczema may be caused by solar light, especially reflections in the water, or light and heat. It can be caused by friction with clothing materials. And, changes in weather, especially cold winds aggravate and sustain existing eczema. Occupational eczema of the hands develops from uses of turpentine, gasoline, alcohol, kerosene and contacts with acids and alkalis, as well as harsh soaps. The familiar "dish-pan hands" is the housewife's form of eczema. And external eczema has been known to develop around the wedding ring when the wife has been guilty of extramarital infidelities. The skin disorder is the outward sign of her inner consciousness of self-imposed guilt. Also the manipulatory sex finger of the male often becomes involved under similar circumstances.

Distinguishing between the different types of eczema is extremely important in their prognosis and treatment. It is certainly a skin condition which requires professional medical attention. Some patients suffering from eczema are apparently in good health, therefore constitutional treatment is not indicated. This is particularly true of the localized types. But, in many other cases where the disease has subsisted for a long duration and various portions of the skin are affected, the general health of the patient may be subnormal.

It is most important to remove all sources of local irritation and all known factors which might produce a contact dermatitis. Patients have known to be allergic to everything under the sun—even some husbands to their wives, and wives to their husbands! Cosmetics affect different people radically and one girl's lipstick may make her mouth beautiful and produce a swollen lip in another. While the removal of a patient from one locale to another can affect the patient's state of health because the change in climate and differences in flora which affect the individual may be apparent, *eczema occurs in all regions.*

Neurogenic and neuro-psychiatric factors do have an evident role in the occurrence of eczema and the care. A parent of a child suffering from eczema must know that the child should get proper rest; regularity of habits and avoidance of overexertion, either mental or physical, are also important. A child with eczema usually tends to be brighter than the average child and therefore tends to want to do more, but the care and cure lies in forcing the child to do less. Often the easing up in scholastic activities will be the cure in infant and adolescent eczema.

Most patients suffering from eczema are concerned about their appearance. The conviction that they must be repulsive to others reinforces their melancholy seclusiveness. "I don't care to go out." "I can't stand the look of repulsion on other people's faces." "I feel self-conscious." "It's not polite to scratch in public where people can see you." Many patients feel dirty (and bathe to excess, thereby increasing the itchiness) and many uninformed patients fear having a contagious or inherited disease—many erroneously believe their eczema is a form of a syphilis inherited from some remote ancestor and visited unto the "third and fourth generation." Embarrassing comments in barber shops, beauty parlors, upon the dance floor or among one's peers can cause a victim to withdraw completely from social contacts. Yet eczema does not drive its victims to ultimate desperation. Few ever attempt suicide.

Anxiety and guilt may be roused by the secondary effects of the disease on others. The housewife who cannot put her hands in water may suffer when she sees her husband obliged to bathe the baby, or the husband may feel guilt as he watches his wife remove ointment stains from his pillow case or scabs from the carpet.

There is no question that the treatment of eczema patients is baffling and often very discouraging, even to a dermatologist. An ointment which may work wonders for one person's skin may not suit the skin of another and may even aggravate the skin of the original patient when the disease recurs at a later date. The patient must realize that dietetic and allergic conditions alter constantly. The doctor himself is very often working in the dark and cooperation with the patient is most important. Many eczema sufferers hasten to run from one skin specialist to another, try one skin ointment after another, but usually any successful change in doctor or remedy is short-lived. Hospitalization often affects a temporary cure which disappears when the patient returns to the outside world. The answers are rather obvious—hospitalized, the patient is removed from allergic conditions and from cumbersome pressures which aggravate his condition and, emotionally, the daily applications of compresses and ointments to an eczema patient is analgous to the early recollections of infancy when he was patted, rubbed, caressed and cared for with tender loving hands.

That the most commonplace distribution of eczema is on the face and arms is of some psychiatric significance. Your skin is the organ of interpersonal contact; and contact with its implied sense of security has been shown to be the psychodynamic need of eczematous individuals. In exhibiting his eczema the patient adopts the position of the supplicant and the weeping of his eczema, like the weeping of a small child, reinforces his appeal. This "open speech" of his skin predates to a period before the eczema sufferer knew how to express his emotions in words. The tendency of eczema patients is to fall into two categories, the "unwanted" and the "spoiled." Dermatologists need to emphasize the importance of psychic adjustment, as well as an understanding of hereditary factors and constitutional allergies of the eczema sufferer. Since in its sundry phases eczema constitutes such a large portion of the dermatologist's medical practice, better understanding among the lay and medical world cannot be overemphasized.

Your doctor must know in detail your social, occupational, sexual and marital world before he can begin to attempt the cure of your eczema. There is no miracle cure; eczema is a study of constant care.

ACNE VULGARIS

A famous dermatologist, S. Rothman, once aptly observed, "One must remember and consider most seriously those diseases which do not end life but which ruin it."

Of all skin diseases acne is particularly pernicious because it occurs at such a bad time—a bad time for patient and a bad time for his family. It comes at a time when the human being is most insecure, most labile in his emotions and when he is trying to find his niche in the world—socially, economically, sexually.

It comes at the very worst time of life because of its impact upon the disposition, the personality, emotions and psyche of the individual concerned. Acne appears at exactly the very moment when personal appearance is of paramount importance. Later in life one's success does not depend so very much on personal appearance, but the adolescent is very dependent upon his appearance. And the exacerbations of acne, the pimples, occur not only at unpredictable times, but apparently at the most inopportune moments. The pimples burst through just at the moment when the boy is having his interview to get into a school, to be admitted to a fraternity, or on a date with the girl he has selected as the target for romance. For the girl going to a very special party, acne seems to break forth with an almost malevolent strength. And acne strikes in the very worst locations, the face, and the shoulders.

Acne is not only a very disturbing disease but it is also one upon which accurate statistics cannot be assembled. Much of it goes unattended by physicians and the customary cases of care are in the young girl patients—largely because the beauty of the young girl is considered of greater importance, and the first signs of the disease are often associated with the girl's first menstrual periods.

Actually, acne occurs in its maximum prevalence among teenagers, the age of Booth Tarkington's classic *Seventeen;* and, contrary to popular belief until 1931, when Dr. Bruno Spock made public his study, the prevalence was greater among males than females and the disease was more severe among males. This fact is due probably to the greater growth of hair on the male face and body at puberty; and that testosterone is likely to be a stronger acnegenic than progesterone. This fact is substantiated by the common occurrence of acne conditions among women and girls using the Pill. Many find themselves victimized by typical adolescent pimply skin (plus superfluous hair and pigmentated "mask of pregnancy" spots), although the Pill is frequently and paradoxically utilized in the treatment of the same condition.

Acne is also a ruinous disease in that certain ideas associated with the disease are "bugaboos" fixed in the lay mind. Somehow since the beginning of time and the first appearance of the disease it has been associated erroneously with ideas of dirt, contagions, sexual aberrations (either excessive or abstinences or inadequacies) and with faulty or filthy habits of all kinds. For years, acne was regarded by many people as an outward sign of masturbatory habits, and the appearance of the bad skin revealed to the outward world the most secret performance of the human individual—more secret, until the publication of *Portnoy's Complaint,* than the act of defecation. This misunderstanding has led, and unfortunately still continues to lead, to terrible conflicts between parents and children, more than with any other disease.

It is quite customary, even today, for an adolescent to be dragged into a doctor's office with a bad case of acne accompanied not only by parents, but by grandparents and a host of other friends and relatives. They are all-too-often guilt ridden. The parents are accusing the child of either doing something wrong or not doing something he should have. The parents will inform the doctor that the skin condition is because the adolescent is either sleeping too much, or not sleeping enough, eating the wrong foods, drinking too many Cokes, or bathing too much or not bathing. The hidden accusation of nocturnal masturbation is undercurrent in many of the interviews and then the child, observing the parent's skin scarred from acne, turns accusingly and reprimands the parent for transferring this same bad skin condition onto another generation. The side-effects of the disease are more malicious than the disease itself for it creates tensions and situations which tend to stretch the existing generation gap to wider areas. The open discussions of sex and sexual relationships are still by-passed and the once beautiful child, now afflicted with ugly purple acne sores, is an unsightly figure in the parents' eyes. A revulsion sets in where love, affection and desire to touch and pet once existed. To the parent who was never bothered with acne the appearance in a child can offer serious emotional disturbances. More tears, tensions and outbursts of misunderstanding occur in doctor's offices with acne than with any other disease.

Acne is also a somato-psychic disease of tremendous proportions, for it affects the mind, the mentality and the personality of the individual almost beyond recall. When one considers that acne is a disease which can last for a decade or more, and for ten or so of the most important and formative years of the psyche, one can easily see how it is capable of leaving permanent scars, not only on the skin itself, but on the *id* of the individual.

So seriously do doctors regard acne and its proper treatment that a colleague of mine summed it up in these words, "If I can save one young boy or girl from the agony of damaging acne, I will feel that my study and practice of medicine has been justified."

Fortunately today the treatment of acne has advanced more than any other dermatological disease. Doctors can keep *acne juveniles* under control and keep the individuals presentable during those extremely vulnerable years from thirteen to twenty-three (only a very small proportion of acne remains clinically active after the twenties). The most important fact of acne must be explained to the patient and to the parent of the patient. Because of the "miracle" shots many parents believe that acne can be cured up overnight and do not take the time or make the effort to encourage, not the *cure,* but the *care* of the disease through the critical years. The best thing your doctor can do is to administer treatment from every practical point of view and again to hit at every link which might be identified with the disease.

First, acne presents a serious cosmetic problem: a severe case with cysts, crusts and discolorations that can cover a patient's face and can be a dreadful cross to bear. As bad as this is in the case of a young man, it is formidably dangerous in the case of a young girl.

Then, especially since our national involvement with the war in Viet Nam, we doctors see many examples of tropical acne where the back of the soldier is mutilated to the degree of being unable to serve in the Armed Forces and possibly being subjected to recurrent *acne vulgaris* throughout a lifetime. Here the disease affects the sexual life of the individual, for although the juvenile face acne may have disappeared, this form is obvious to a spectator either on the beach or in the intimacy of sexual contact. In the latter case, many a sex partner has been "turned off" for life—turned off, tragically, by someone who might have been a logical choice as a sex partner in every other respect.

The cures which are available under medical direction include the use of systemic antibacterial agents and the administration of certain hormones—in girls estrogenic hormones in proper dosages before the menses are safe and sometimes effective.

In the care of acne there are a number of correlating links such as tension, fatigue and the psyche involved. It has often been referred to as an American adolescent disease, as it seems to be more prevalent in America than in any other section of the world. Some doctors have identified it with the overindulgence of the American teenager, especially in dietary habits. (It is an accepted fact that excessive use of chocolate—because of its content of bromides—can, in many cases, aggravate an acne condition.) The fact is, acne is serious and damaging. And, one of its most damaging aspects is the scarring which follows acne. Interestingly enough, the scarring by acne does not necessarily go along with the severity of the acne, and it is not necessarily an obligatory sequence. There seems to exist a tendency among some people to scar with skin lesions and others not to scar.

What can be done about acne scarring? The treatment is in the hands of the individual dermatologist. Usually the treatment of scarring is peeling, superficially with dry ice, phenol, resorcinol, to the very deepest form which is called dermabrasion or plastic planing. The methods used are entirely up to patient and doctor relative to the seriousness of the scarring.

In the treatment of acne the most important fact to know is that it is a skin disease which can be managed and helped in most cases. It is also a disease in which the patient and the physicians and the patient's family should remember at all times, the beginning of acne in the young boy or girl should not be dismissed as just the appearance of a few teenage pimples which will disappear in time and be of little or no consequence; it's not a case where nothing can be done and need be done; it is not to be dismissed as nature's way of indicating one of the commonplace "growing pains" to which man is subject.

No case of pimples, however mild, should be ignored or treated with commercially advertised "cosmetic cures" (for they very often exaggerate the acne). Doctors might suggest a product such as Liquimat for covering acne lesions. It is easily applied and quite satisfactory for temporary use. The sensitive young boy or girl should be examined and the reasons for his or her acne investigated. While some may be from the customary cause of puberal growth of glands and hair follicles, other causes might be dietary, or internal infections.

A great deal needs to be done for the adolescent affected with acne, and a great deal *can* be done for almost every sufferer today if the disease is tended to in time.

ROSACEA

Acne rosacea—or flushing acne—is more common in women than in men, and usually occurs in those in their forties and fifties. The two essential symptoms are an increased vascularity and a tendency to form papules on the blush areas of the cheeks, the chin, the nose, the middle of the forehead and the V-shaped space at the top of the bosom.

It was Mark Twain who observed that, "Man is the only animal that blushes—or has need to . . ." The ingestion of hot or alcoholic drinks, too much coffee or tea, or heavily seasoned and highly spiced foods, and the taking of hurried meals may produce considerable change in the facial appearance of a rosacea sufferer, and it is possible that the stomach provokes the condition.

The flushing which is due to menopause has long been attributed to endocrine disturbance. Flushing, if dependent upon emotion, is usually associated with intense excitement of joy or anger.

> "Sudden a thought came like a full blown rose,
> Flushing his brow, and in his pained heart
> Made purple riot."
>
> —John Keats, "The Eve of St. Agnes"

Psychiatric examination of patients suffering from rosacea would indicate that some of them have had extreme emotional problems before the onset of the skin disease. Social anxiety seems to be the handmaiden of patients with rosacea. Many have embarrassment over social conversation; they are "shy," and like to be in the background. Almost uniformly, rosacea patients relate that "excitement and worry," among other factors, bring on "hot flashes" which accompany the disease. Problems of sociality and sexuality aggravate the condition. (A movie with Doris Day and Cary Grant evolved around a girl who suffered from rosacea, and presented a humorous incident revolving around a situation which is rarely funny and often very emotionally disturbing, but not uncommon.)

The blushing which is another phase of rosacea results from feelings of shame, modesty or confusion. One patient confessed to me that her blushing commenced when she first began masturbating at an early age and upon waking and joining her schoolmates she felt soiled, dirty, and isolated. She began to suspect that they and her teachers knew what she had been doing and the blush on her face was the physical evidence of her masturbatory habits. She felt that the entire world knew her personal habits and weaknesses, and her rosacea became the barrier between herself and the outside world by the time she was in her early twenties.

Amazingly, the situations which produce rosacea are commonplace and fortunately do not affect most people (although most individuals suffer an attack of vasomotor instability of the "butterfly" region of the cheeks and bridge of the nose at one time or another in a lifetime). The persons who are more frequently affected are patients who display a dependence upon the opinion of others, have the compulsive desire to please, the constant fear of attracting attention. The patient is usually a victim of unusually strong feelings of guilt, shame and inferiority. Blushing, strangely enough, is compatible with complete innocence or modesty.

> "Full many a flower is born to blush unseen,
> And waste its sweetness on the desert air."

So wrote Gray in "Elegy Written in a Country Churchyard." He gives us the portrait of an innocent maiden to whom sexuality was a frightening experience, one for whom death was preferable. Actually, blushing occurs most typically in individuals in whom there is a conflict between morality and natural sexual impulses. The blushes occur disastrously at certain periods in life: either before the female is ready for actual sexual encounter but has dreamed and imagined them in degrees which leave her guilt-laden, or after her female functions for childbearing have ceased to exist and she is embarrassed to think that she still has "carnal" desires. In actuality both situations are illogical, but nevertheless quite real to the patient. They are hangovers from Victorian morality which still shreds a grey pall over a large part of human life.

Physiologically, rosacea is a tendency to lose contractile power of the smaller blood vessels of the face, but emotional factors are of fundamental importance in most cases of rosacea. The disease is affected by emotional disturbances which can produce a permanent blush or can create gastric tones which lead to a permanent flush. The appearance of blushing and flushing of the skin is quite apparent in many psychoneurotic patients. For in neuroses, the skin is very often the target of self-punishment, self-castration, self-destruction and self-contamination and -infestation. Naturally, the obvious blush or flush of guilt would be a significant manifestation of an inner emotional disturbance.

The treatment by the dermatologist is directed in two channels: 1) the avoidance of those conditions which create the vasomotor flushing and 2) measure of lessening sebaceous hyperactivity.

ERYTHEMA SIMPLEX

Erythema simplex is a redness of the skin—actually more a symptom than a disease—diffused over wide areas or circumscribed patches, and due to the increased flow of peripheral blood.

The causes of the disease are varied, the most common being exposure to extremes of temperature, physical injury, sensitivity to drugs, and fever.

There is no thickening of the skin and the redness disappears momentarily on pressure. Itching and burning, alone or in combination, may be associated with this phenomenon.

Erythema simplex occurs in many and varied disorders; it is essential to determine the cause before attempting to apply other than palliative treatment measures.

PRURITUS (ITCHING)

Strictly speaking, *pruritus* is another symptom, and one of the most common of complaints: a sensation, generalized or localized, which one instinctively attempts to relieve by scratching the skin in the affected area.

Basically, itching is caused by mildly irritant stimuli which act on the epidermal nerve endings for *pain.* No specific stimulus is required. Both the peripheral and the central threshholds for itching may vary considerably among different people and in the same person at different times. Everyone experiences a moderate transitory pruritus at times—this is physiologic. It is only when itching is persistent and troublesome that it becomes pathologic.

Secondary pruritus occurs in most skin diseases (although, in characteristic cases, not in such things as syphilis or psoriasis), and is especially severe in scabies, pediculosis, insect bites, hives, eczema, contact dermatitis, food allergy dermatitis and prickly heat.

It may be the sole sign, however, of a serious systemic

disease. It thus demands careful evaluation—evaluation which is more than skin deep, because the itching may be caused by diabetes mellitus, nephritis, disease of the liver and gall bladder, cancer, leukemia, tuberculosis, gout, hardening of the arteries, and thyroid problems. Other causative factors can include pregnancy, the change of life, infection, and drug or food allergy. Itching may also be psychosomatic.

Scratching complicates the condition and should be avoided as much as possible. Areas of redness, wheals, excoriated papules, fissures, and crusts may be produced. Secondary infection may occur. In prolonged itching and scratching, thickening and increased pigmentation of the skin frequently ensue.

For treatment, it is essential to find and remove the cause of the itching. Your physician should be consulted. All medicaments should be stopped, *if this is feasible*—those being used either internally or externally. Many drugs in common use may produce a reaction, as may home remedies. Rough surfaces or woolen clothing should be avoided. Environmental temperature changes should be minimized.

Soothing baths are advisable in extensive pruritus. Baths from ten to twenty minutes twice a day in a tubful of lukewarm water containing one-half to one cup of cooked (therefore soluble) cornstarch, with the application afterwards of a bland antipruritic preparation like calamine lotion or witch hazel, can often help. Other remedies should be prescribed by your physician to avoid the possibility of sensitivity reactions.

Relief or arrest of any underlying disease, plus symptomatic therapy, will usually relieve the distress.

MILIARIA (HEAT RASH)

This is an acute inflammatory dermatitis due to keratin obstruction of the sweat ducts. The disease is most common in infants, in the obese, and in those exposed to excessive heat and humidity for long periods of time. Following profuse sweating, closely grouped papules and vesiculopapules appear on an erythematous base—associated with itching and burning.

Areas most commonly affected are the chest, back, waistline, and skin folds. The inflammation subsides in a few days and may be followed by a surface peeling of the skin. Recurrent attacks are common, however, and in prolonged cases the sweating mechanism may become impaired (a condition frequently seen in the tropics, with occasional complete inability to sweat, followed by severe weakness and lassitude). Heat rash must be distinguished from seborrheic dermatitis, contact dermatitis, secondary syphilis, drug eruption, and id conditions.

Treatment consists in keeping the patient as cool as possible and avoiding those conditions which promote perspiration. Baths containing starch are soothing. Calamine lotion will frequently relieve itching. See your physician if the condition persists.

INTERTRIGO (CHAFING)

Chafing is the term for a superficial inflammation (acute) of apposing skin surfaces. It is characterized by erythema, abrasion, maceration and, in some cases, superficial fissuring. Moisture, warmth and the friction of two apposing skin surfaces rubbing together—these factors cause the condition known as chafing. An infection, either bacterial or mycotic, almost invariably ensues as a complication.

Areas most likely to be affected include the armpits, the groins, the anal region, the interdigital spaces of the hands and feet, and the area beneath the breasts. Obesity and hot weather are important predisposing factors. Burning and itching are common.

Preventative measures include proper cleansing and the continued use of a dusting powder (in moderate amounts so as to avoid caking), and in those who are overweight, reducing. Wear cool, well aerated clothing and avoid strenous activity in hot weather, if this is possible.

SEBORRHEIC DERMATITIS (CRADLE CAP, DANDRUFF)

This is an acute or subacute inflammatory disease which originates in those areas most profusely supplied by sebaceous glands—especially the scalp, eyebrows, wings of the nose, areas behind the ears, mid-chest and mid-back, arm pits, and groins. It is characterized by superficial, irregularly sized and shaped pink or slightly red patches, covered with greasy yellowish or dry white, brawny scales (*e.g.* dandruff).

The underlying casual factor in the oily type is increased activity of the sebaceous glands (*seborrhea* is often most pronounced during puberty). Oily areas provide excellent sites for bacterial or fungous growth or both. Seborrhea seems definitely related to endocrine changes (disturbed androgen—estrogen balance) and yet there are also such etiologic possibilities as heredity, excess ingestion of fat and carbohydrates (including alcohol), gastrointestinal disturbance, fatigue, excessive perspiration, poor personal hygiene, climatic conditions, and emotional factors.

The symptoms and signs include the elementary lesions which are very red macules or papules about the hair follicles which may merge. Several body areas may be involved simultaneously.

Diagnosis must exclude syphilids, contact dermatitis, pityriasis rosea, atopic eczema, superimposed fungous infections, and psoriasis.

The acute dermatitis ordinarily responds within a few days or weeks to treatment, while the subacute or chronic types may be extremely refractory. Treatment should be prescribed by a physician who chooses medicaments according to the clinical stage of the eruption and the regions involved: hairy, intertriginous, or glabrous (hairless) skin. Erythema, edema, and vesiculation generally characterize the acute stage; oozing, crusting and scaling, the subacute; pigmentary changes, thickening and fissuring, the chronic.

General measures include regular rest and sleeping periods; frequent bathing; use of soap substitutes, as soap is irritating; high protein, low carbohydrate, low fat diet; weight reduction, if indicated; prohibition of alcohol; vitamin B complex; injections of crude liver extract fortified with pyridoxine; elimination of possible contact allergens—medicaments, perfumes, deodorants, clothing, dyes, nail polish, metals (nickel in costume jewelry); and eradication of areas of infection.

SEBACEOUS CYST (WEN)

A sebaceous cyst is a slow-growing benign cystic tumor of the skin which results from occlusion of the sebaceous gland ducts, and frequently is found on the scalp, ears, face, back, or scrotum.

On palpation, the cystic mass is firm, globular, movable, and if not infected, nontender. It seldom causes any discomfort. Sebaceous cysts should be differentiated from lipomas and other tumors, malignant and benign, late stages of syphilis, inflamed lymph nodes, and so forth.

The treatment of choice is surgical excision of the intact tumor. Incision and drainage, followed by electrocautery of the inner surface of the sac of the cyst, has been successful in many cases. Recurrence is inevitable if the capsule is not completely removed or destroyed.

IMPETIGO

Impetigo is a common contagious skin infection, whose lesions are characterized by thin-walled vesicles, pustules, and thick superficial crusts. Streptococcal and staphylococcal infections of the superficial skin is responsible. Poor hygiene, overcrowding, and faulty diet are predisposing factors. Impetigo is most prevalent in hot, moist climates. A scratch, abrasion or some other such damage to the integrity of the skin is generally necessary as a portal of entry to the skin. It usually occurs in infants and children—becoming readily epidemic in institutions such as hospitals and orphanages. The newborn are especially susceptible.

Unless complicated by constitutional systems, impetigo can be relived in three to ten days by effective treatment; without treatment the course is unpredictable. If you suspect this skin disease, consult your physician. He is the one to distinguish the pustules and crusts with their thin straw-colored discharge from secondary syphilis and drug eruptions, for example. He will first remove the crusts and tops of the vesicles, vesicopustules and bullae before attempting local treatment. This is the first and most important step. Further treatment will vary and should not be attempted by the layman.

FURUNCLE AND CARBUNCLE

Furuncle—or boil—is a tender, acute inflammatory nodule which becomes a pustule with discharging, a central core of necrotic tissue and a variable amount of bloody, pussy discharge. The lesions are apt to be multiple and may occur anywhere on the skin, but are more apt to be found on the neck, armpits, breast, extremities, face and ear. Lesions within the external auditory canal and the nose, and on the central part of the face are often painful and a cause for great concern.

A *carbuncle* is a multiple abcess characterized by sloughing at numerous points on the surface. The lesion resembles a furuncle except for being larger, flatter, denser, less rapidly developed, and more painful. It may be accompanied by severe constitutional symptoms (prostration, somnolence, stupor). It is most frequently seen in men, often occurring on the nape of the neck, and may be either superficial or deep. It is followed by extensive sloughs, ulcers, and large scars. Furuncles and small carbuncles should be protected from irritation, and moist heat should be applied intermittently. The skin should be kept clean by frequent washing with soap and water. A physician may recommend X-ray treatments. Ointments and antibiotics may be prescribed.

ERYSIPELAS

This is an acute infection of the skin caused by a streptococcus and characterized by a sharply demarcated, red, swollen area, with accompanying fever and malaise.

The same type of streptococcus may cause scarlet fever, and other streptococcal diseases. This skin disease is more prevalent during the winter and early spring and most common among older people.

The onset of *erysipelas* is ordinarily characterized by chills, fever, nausea and vomiting a day or so before the skin lesions appear. However, the lesions may develop without these symptoms. In facial erysipelas, a characteristic "butterfly" appearance is frequent, due to symmetrical distribution of the process, beginning at the bridge of the nose and extending over the cheeks.

Temperatures as high as 105° may accompany the spread of the lesion. If untreated, the skin becomes a shiny reddish purple on the fourth or fifth day and the swelling begins to subside. Desquamation, especially loose scales peeling away, begins in about a week.

Isolation is recommended if at all possible and bed and body clothing should be disinfected. Bed rest and a high protein, high vitamin, bland diet with liberal amounts of fluids are helpful. Sulfonamides and penicillin have tremendously improved the prognosis of erysipelas, but these should only be used under the care of your doctor.

HERPES SIMPLEX (FEVER BLISTER)

Fever blisters are caused by a virus; the infection is characterized by the formation of groups of small blisters, individual or multiple, filled with clear fluid on slightly raised inflammatory bases.

A medium-sized virus is the infecting agent. It is presumed that this virus remains dormant in the skin, only to be stimulated to activity by overexposure to sunlight, menstruation, fever, emotional stress, ingestion of certain foods, or the like. The ordeal of dental work can also trigger an outbreak, as can the trauma of sexual intercourse.

Typical lesions develop rapidly, with burning, itching and tingling, and persist for five to ten days; then gradually subside and disappear; sometimes, if frequently recurrent at the same site, there is resultant scarring.

Skin lesions are most common on the face, about the mouth or on the lips, or on the genitals or buttocks. Mucous membrane eruptions occur most frequently as small, whitish plaques or *aphthous ulcers* (canker sores). Herpes of the vagina also appears as plaques or ulcers.

There is no scientific treatment. Symptomatic relief and prevention of secondary infection should be attempted. Skin lesions may be mopped with cotton soaked in 95 percent alcohol, spirits of camphor or benzalkonium chloride, followed by a dusting powder. Hard, dry crusts may be softened by a soothing ointment. Mouth and other mucous membrane lesions may be benefited by a detergent and bactericidal solution.

Canker sores (ulcers), when persistent and painful, may be touched with a silver nitrate stick or a swab dipped in 19 percent silver nitrate solution followed by thorough rinsing with water. Eye lesions should be treated by an ophthalmologist. Chronic recurrent cases may be benefited by X-ray therapy administered by one experienced in its use.

WARTS

Warts are induced by a filtrable virus. The disease is readily transmitted among persons in close association, although the factors that predispose one to infection are not well known. The incubation period varies from three weeks to several months.

Warts occur most commonly on the hand, less frequently on the sole of the foot, the face and the genitalia. Warts have a characteristic pebbly, cauliflower-like surface, on which thrombosed blood vessels appear as black dots. Warts may become depressed below the surface, in areas where there is pressure such as the sole of the foot. These are known as plantar warts, or *papillomas.*

Some warts disappear spontaneously; others persist for years. Specific treatment is available only for *condylomata acuminata* (venereal warts) and consists of podophyllin carefully applied to each lesion with an applicator stick.

Consult your physician before attempting to remove warts. Care should be taken not to use a treatment so vigorously as to leave a scar.

CUTANEOUS TUBERCULOSIS

This term refers to any skin lesion due to *mycotuberculosis,* either directly by local infection, or indirectly from infection elsewhere in the body. About 85 percent of the cases are caused by the human type of tubercle bacillus, the remainder by the bovine type. The disease is relatively rare in the United States. While it may be seen in tuberculous children or adolescents, it occurs most frequently in persons in the lower income groups living under unhygienic conditions.

The skin lesions frequently are associated with tuberculous lesions elsewhere, and the basic pathology is similar to that of tuberculosis generally.

All the therapeutic measures for tuberculosis apply equally well in cutaneous tuberculosis and only a few special procedures are necessary. These should be prescribed by a qualified physician.

SCABIES (THE ITCH)

The itch is a highly contagious parasitic skin disease. It is characterized by burrows in the skin, multiform eruptions, and intense itching that occurs chiefly at night.

Scabies is caused by the itch mite. It is acquired through intimate contact with an infested individual or infested clothing. Most prevalent among persons living under crowded, unhygienic conditions, infestation often involves an entire household.

The impregnanted female itch mite burrows into the horny layer of the skin and deposits her eggs. These hatch within four to eight days, emerge, and travel across the skin to enter the hair follicles. Itching is most intense at night because of the nocturnal activity of the parasites. The characteristic lesion is the burrow, which appears as a fine wavy dark line.

Treatment is entirely external. It involves a course of cleansing of the body and clothing, and the application of medication. Sulfur ointment is the time-honored antiscabetic medicament.

ATOPIC DERMATITIS (See: Eczema)

This is a chronic superficial inflammation of the skin characterized by thickening, excoriation, and lichenification,* with associated itching. It often begins in infancy and usually occurs in individuals with a high family incidence of allergic diseases.

Basically, it is allergic in origin, with a strong hereditary factor. Neurocirculatory and emotional instability are frequent predisposing factors. Numerous allergens have been found to be responsible—foods such as chocolate, oranges, strawberries and tomatoes; contactants such as wool, cotton, paint, cosmetics, oils. Inhalants (*e.g.* dander, pollen, dust) also frequently are responsible.

Itching, usually worse at night, is the outstanding subjective symptom. Papules with excoriated and crusted tops are the primary cutaneous lesions.

Usually, although not always, atopic dermatitis begins in early infancy and continues with a history of alternating allergic diseases into adulthood.

Those suffering from atopic dermatitis should be taught to avoid emotional upsets as much as possible. Contact with irritants should be avoided. A physician can often locate the

* *Lichenification*—Thickening of the skin and increase of its markings by a gathering together or grouping of papules. Lichens are forms of plant life, fungus and algae. The word is used for those designated dermatoses which resemble botanical formations.

cause of the condition by varying tests; he can also prescribe medication to allay itching.

PITYRIASIS ROSEA

This inflammatory disease of the skin is of unknown origin and characterized by maculosquamous lesions.

A herald patch often appears about seven to ten days before the generalized eruption. This is a rose- or fawn-colored, well-demarcated, oval or circinate patch covered by a dry scale. By the time it has increased in diameter and perhaps begun to fade, similar lesions appear on the trunk, buttocks, or extremities.

The disease is self-limited. Without treatment, it may persist for six to eight weeks—occasionally much longer. With appropriate treatment, the course can be considerably shortened. Recovery without permanent residual effects is the rule. Recurrences are rare.

LUPUS ERYTHEMATOSUS

This is a relatively rare systemic disease, characterized by cutaneous lesions which consist of scaling patches of various sizes and result in superficial atrophy of the skin, and scar formation.

The cause is unknown. The disease is more common in women than in men, usually occuring in the thirties. The first attack frequently follows over-exposure to the sun.

There is both a mild, local and a severe, generalized form

of *lupus erythematosus,* considered by many to be completely separate disease entities. Their skin manifestations must be distinguished from such diseases as seborrheic dermatitis, psoriasis of the face and scalp, acne rosacea, and late syphilis. In the chronic form of the skin disease, the course of the disease is capricious—atrophy and scarring may or may not occur, but once atrophy has appeared, treatment may be directed towards destruction of the lesions. In any case, your physician will recommend a thorough physical examination to determine the type of lupus, the systemic type frequently occurring without any evidence in the skin. There will be a search for possible foci of infection, and he will select the best time for the eradication of these foci. In chronic lupus erythematosus, this may be done immediately; in the acute and subacute forms the focus of infection must not be tampered with until a period of remission.

Rest, avoidance of overwork and supportive care are extremely important in the treatment of all forms of this disease. Further treatment should be under the direction of your physician. He may prescribe carbon dioxide snow for topical application to chronic lesions, possibly antibiotics or steroids in the acute and subacute forms.

SCLERODERMA

This chronic localized or diffuse skin disease, of unknown etiology, is characterized by fibrosis, rigidity, and atrophy of the skin and subcutaneous tissues.

Scleroderma is most common in women during middle life. The onset usually is gradual. The skin becomes smooth and shiny and the face assumes a masklike appearance. The disease usually progresses slowly, with periods of remission. Spontaneous recovery has been observed, however, particularly among children.

Although there is no evidence that the disorder is due to nutritional deficiency, a balanced diet—preferably with general vitamin supplementation—should be maintained. Your physician may prescribe medication to cause regression of lesions and increase muscular strength. Measures to soften the skin and improve blood supply may be useful: massage, warm baths, bland ointments.

CORN

A *corn* is a circumscribed, cone-shaped hypertrophy of the epidermis, the apex of which presses on the corium. Corns result from persistent trauma to the skin. Ill-fitting footwear is a common cause of corns of the feet.

Corns are pea-size or larger lesions, have a whitish center, and are spontaneously painful, especially with change of weather. *Hard* corns occur on the prominent protuberances of the foot and especially the toes. *Soft* corns occur between the toes and, because of the moisture and maceration, are whiter and softer.

Avoidance of the offending trauma will cure most cases of corns. Activity may be changed and the manner in which it is performed. A change in footwear, with the footwear designed to distribute the pressure more evenly, is essential to a lasting cure.

There are various softening and destructive agents which

will give temporary relief or hasten cure. A corn plaster may give temporary relief. To soften the lesions they may be soaked in hot water to which soap has been added. Care must be taken especially in diabetics not to cause bleeding or infection. Your physician may prescribe the use of other softening or destructive agents.

DECUBITUS (BED SORE, PRESSURE SORE)

This is a local necrosis (death) of the skin and subcutaneous tissues overlying a bony prominence which has been subjected to prolonged pressure against an external object (*e.g.* bed, cast, splint). It is most frequently seen in patients long bed ridden.

The essential cause is local pressure upon the tissues. The partial or complete occlusion of blood supply leads to necrosis and gangrene. First, the more sensitive subcutaneous and deeper tissues are damaged, and later the skin becomes necrotic. Pressure combined with injury to the skin from ill-adjusted supports or wrinkled bed covers or clothing may cause small breaks in the skin through which infection is introduced.

Three stages of *decubitus* are recognized: threatened, inevitable and ulcer. Threatened decubitus is indicated by a redness of the skin which disappears when pressure is applied. The skin and tissues are still soft. An inevitable decubitus is diagnosed by the presence of redness, unaffected by digital pressure. Ulcer is characterized by tissue necrosis.

Prevention is the most effective form of treatment. Frequent change of posture and redistribution of points of contact. Bed linens should be kept taut and clean and free from wrinkles or small, hard particles. The patient's skin should be kept dry and clean at all times. Dressings should be changed frequently.

Malnutrition is an important causative factor in decubitus. To restore the nitrogen balance from negative to positive—a high protein, high caloric diet is needed.

Threatened decubitus requires forceful employment of all the prophylactic measures; stimulation of the circulation by gentle massage may be done. Inevitable decubitus and ulcer may be treated conservatively or surgically. Surgical intervention greatly reduces healing time.

NEVI (MOLES, BEAUTY SPOTS, BIRTHMARKS)

Many cutaneous diseases can be included under the term *nevus.* Only the common ones are discussed here.

The term in general refers to circumscribed, benign new growths of the skin that occur as the result of congenital maldevelopment or as later hyperplasia of embryonal rests.

Freckles and "Liver Spots"

These, not moles per se, are both collections (abnormal) of pigment, which are small and circumscribed in the case of freckles and larger and more diffuse in liver spots. The color may be various shades of brown—even black. Freckles usually develop in childhood in areas exposed to sunlight. Liver spots have a variety of causes, including heat and irritation and sometimes in connection with various diseases. Local therapy, which often is unsatisfactory, consists of the application of bleaching cream. Also, they may be removed by the application of dry ice or certain acidic substances so as to remove just the superficial layers of the skin.

Hyperkeratotic and Verrucose Nevi

These occur anywhere on the body and may be various shades of brown. They may be of a linear distribution or may assume a variety of patterns. They don't often disappear; they rarely become malignant. If feasible and desired, surgical excision is possible.

Pigmented Nevi

These may occur anywhere on the body. The color may vary from light brown to slate blue. They may be hairy or hairless, flat or elevated, and vary in size. In general, the flat, smooth, hairless, deeply pigmented nevus has more tendency to become malignant. This is especially true on the lower extremities. It is felt by some that any nevus can become malignant, and that constant trauma, irritation and inadequate removal predispose to such malignant changes.

Nevi containing hairs, especially soft nevi, rarely undergo malignant transformation. Indications for removal are cosmetic. If feasible and desired, surgical excision is possible. Pigmented nevi are frequently confused with freckles or liver spots, the latter having nothing to do with the liver. Pigmented nevi disappear only rarely without therapy. If there is anything unusual about a nevus, expert opinion should be sought.

HEMANGIOMAS

Hemangiomas, localized hyperplasias of the blood vascular tissue of the skin, include:

Flat Angioma (Port-Wine Mark)

This is a macular, superficial hemangioma which can occur on any part of the body. It does not become malignant and is not affected by radiotherapy or any local treatment. It can be disguised to some extent by covering with a cosmetic cream.

Cavernous Angioma (Strawberry Mark)

A nodular, soft angiomatous mass, fairly deep-seated, which blanches on pressure. It may occur anywhere but is common on the face and neck. Such angiomas are present at birth or soon thereafter. Usually, they disappear without active therapy in a few years. They do not become malignant. The various types of therapy include repeated application of solid carbon dioxide, X-ray treatments, radium, and injection of sclerosing solution. Treatment should be started early in infancy. Some of these lesions tend to disappear spontaneously.

Stellate Angioma (Spider Nevus)

An angioma consisting of a central point from which numerous telangiectatic vessels radiate in a star fashion. The lesions may occur anywhere on the body, but are most frequent on the face. They may be associated with hepatic disease, hypertension, and pregnancy, but can also occur under normal circumstances. Disappearance occurs spontaneously only in pregnancy. These angiomas do not become malignant. Therapy consists of destruction of the central point by electrolysis.

Senile Angioma (Ruby Spot)

A small compressible mass of blood vessels which can develop anywhere on the body of elderly individuals. It is of no significance and requires no therapy.

HYPERIDROSIS AND BROMIDROSIS

Hyperidrosis is overactivity of the sweat glands. Excessive perspiration may be general or confined to the palms, soles, axillas (armpits), inframammory regions, or groin. Sweating of the palms and soles may be psychogenic in origin and the odors accompanying can be quite offensive. The skin in the affected areas is often livid or dusky blue (especially on the soles of the feet). In severe cases, sogginess of the skin, fissuring and scaling (especially on the feet) will occur. Hyperidrosis may be a cause or a contributing factor in the production of various skin diseases such as fungus and infections, contact dermatitis, food allergy and dermatoses and seborrheic dermatitis.

Generalized hyperidrosis frequently accompanies fever or certain systemic diseases such as anemia and diabetes. Obesity and endocrine dysfunction (hyperthyroidism) also may cause generalized sweating. Occasionally, an abnormality or a disease of the nervous system may be the cause.

The reason for localized hyperidrosis is not clear since it usually occurs in otherwise normal individuals. However, the patient may be in a state of overanxiety or hypertension. The bad odor which is evident in *bromidrosis* is caused by decomposition of the sweat and cellular debris by thc action of bacteria and yeasts.

For general hyperidrosis, treatment of the underlying systemic disease or psychotherapy is necessary. The condition is usually somewhat refractory and uncontrolled cases can lead to further complications. Prescribed medication can be given by your dermatologist but the side effects of many of the prescribed medications are annoying.

Aluminum chloride solutions and potassium permanganate compresses can be useful in localized hyperidrosis. Five percent formaldehyde solution may be painted on the soles of the feet or the palm of the hands and allowed to remain overnight, or one can soak the soles and palms in a 5 percent solution of formaldehyde with a quart of lukewarm water; sensitization reactions may result. A drying powder (for example, B.F.I.) should be applied once a day for several days and thereafter as indicated. Psychotherapy may be required before the cure is affected.

The treatment for *bromidrosis* is essentially the same but the response may be more satisfactory. Unpleasant odor of the armpit area is due to the action of bacteria on apocrine sweat; therefore scrupulous cleaning is essential. Shaving the auxillary hair is important in reducing odor. A topical antibiotic such as 5 percent neomycin solution is probably the best deodorant for the axillary region. Bacterial count can also be reduced by a germicidal soap. In extreme cases, removal of the sweat glands in the axillary areas will stop the excessive flow of sweat.

VITILIGO

Loss of pigment—*vitiligo*—usually occurs in sharply demarcated areas of the skin. A few or numerous patches, or (rarely) depigmentation over the entire body may be the pattern observed. A familial history is often present.

The cause of vitiligo is unknown. It may appear at any time up to middle age, and anywhere on the body, though most frequently on the hands and face. The melanocytes are intact, but fail to deposit melanin in the affected epidermal areas. Vitiligo is not a manifestation of a systemic disease; it is a cosmetic defect and particularly disfiguring to black people and to persons whose surrounding skin is highly tanned or dark olive color. The affected areas can be extremely sensitive to sunlight. The depigmented areas may slowly enlarge peripherally. If hairy areas are involved, depigmentation of the hair also occurs. Return of pigment, spontaneously or following treatment, is rare.

A real case of vitiligo must be differentiated from the temporary, secondary depigmentation which is sometimes seen in pityriasis rosea, atopic dermatitis, seborrheic dermatitis or following exposure to antioxidants used in rubber gloves. In these cases pigmentation customarily returns after the inflammation subsides or following cessation of use of the chemical. Differentiation also must be made from diseases causing depigmentation due to atrophy or scarring.

No satisfactory treatment for vitiligo is known. Because the affected areas are sensitive to sunlight, application of a sun-screening product before exposure is advisable. Bleaching of the surrounding skin can be harmful and is most impractical. Staining preparations such as potassium permanganate, walnut-shell extracts and common pigments have not proven satisfactory. Esthetically good results can be obtained by the use of cosmetic pastes or lotions (*i.e.* Covermark), matched and applied by an experienced cosmetic technician.

YOUR DERMATOLOGIST IS A SYPHILOLOGIST

When you enter the office of your dermatologist, you may see, on his wall, a certificate which reads:

Diplomate, American Board of Dermatology & Syphilology

You will probably be somewhat disconcerted unless you are acquainted with the history of dermatology.

Actually, it evolved as a specialized study quite late in the chronology of medicine. The first systematic treatise on skin disease was published *(De Morbis Cutaneis)* in 1572 by Gerolamo Merculaire, but physicians were at that time still confused by the dermatologic manifestations of syphilis, leprosy and small pox and unable to distinguish between a true skin disease and a mere symptom. Modern dermatology began in 1798 with Robert Willan's *Description and Treatment of Cutaneous Diseases.* This book made the doctor the official father of the speciality. He classified primary lesions and he used *colored* illustrations, both facts were of great importance.

The fact that the study of skin diseases was in the beginning so closely linked to the venereal diseases is undoubtedly one of the main reasons why there has ensued so many misundcrstandings, so many taboos among lay people, and such a disinclination among doctors to specialize in the subject.

Today, dermatologists have a 29 percent annual increase in patient census while general practitioners have 10 percent fewer. The growth among the dermatologists was the largest reported. Why?

As we have shown, dermatology today includes many manifestations of skin malady totally disassociated from venereal disease. These diseases, however, do seriously affect the personality of the individual. Though repulsive to the human eye, most are not contagious and very often originate in allergies, or from bacterial infection.

In the beginning, however, there was little question that a skin disease did not carry a connotation of sexual origin. As we all know, it takes centures to eradicate old wive's tales and some never actually disappear from circulation. The combination of guilt and fear and the association of a skin ailment with venereal diseases has led many an innocent victim of acne vulgaris or psoriasis to emotions of total desperation.

The name venereal disease is in itself of common interest, as it is derived from the name of Venus, the Love Goddess and the gifts she bestows are indeed sometimes questionable.

SYPHILIS

It is Sir William Osler who made the profound observation, "To know syphilis is to know medicine!"

Yet today, due to the post World War II decreases in the syphilis rate, many medical students have graduated from medical school without being properly exposed to the oldest scourge of mankind—and the most difficult to conquer. Despite interims of decline, the dread disease is still prevalent and again on the rise.

The controversy over whether syphilis existed in Europe prior to the return of Columbus from his first voyage to the Americas in 1493 will probably never be entirely resolved. There is much evidence of the existence of syphilis in the pre-Columbian skulls discovered in the Americas; there is also some evidence that a type of syphilis had existed in Europe prior to Columbus' first journey. Some authorities tend to believe that syphilis has been with us since the beginning of time, but to authenticate such claims would be difficult. Needless to say, from its first appearance in epidemic numbers it has been the curse of man. Dias de Isla (who is credited with isolating the disease) was practicing in Barcelona when Columbus returned in 1493. He declared the disease was unknown in Spain at that time. Dias credited the source to the sailors on Columbus' ships and named the disease "disease of the Isle of Española." In 1494, King Charles VIII of France invaded Naples with an army composed of mercenary soldiers, many of whom were Spanish, and the disease spread and became known as the disease of Naples. As Charles' army moved over Europe, so travelled the disease. In early historic art relics one finds plaques dedicated to "Triumph of the High and Mighty Dame Syphilis, Queen of the Fountain of Love." From its original appearance, the disease was associated with sexual intercourse and everywhere the disease raised its ugly head it was regarded as new and names for it appeared which attempted to shift the responsibility to others. The Italians called it the Spanish or French disease; the French called it the Italian or Neopolitan disease; the English called it the French disease; the Russians called it the Polish; the Turks called it the French.

Publications soon appeared and the first illustration (a syphilitic kneeling at the fountain of Venus) is attributed to Albert Durer in 1496, although Grunspeck's famous illustration may have appeared also in 1496.

Understanding of the clinical characteristics of syphilis developed early in the sixteenth century and Fracastor, physician and author, named the disease in his poem "Syphilissive Morbus Gallicus," where he writes, "For one small pleasure I suffer a thousand misfortunes." Sexual contact was recognized as the source of syphilis, but unhygenic conditions were also credited with being a source. The disease was clearly differentiated from gonorrhea at first, but in time became confused with gonorrhea. Congenital syphilis, too, was soon recognized.

Paracelsus is given credit for the introduction of mercury as a cure, but mercury was so commonly used in skin ailments that it must have been tried by many physicians. Fever and sweating was in vogue during the seventeenth and eighteenth centuries as cures. In the nineteenth century there lived two great syphilographers, Phillip Ricord and Jean

Alfred Fournier. It is Ricord who is credited with the witticism, "In the beginning God created the Heavens, Earth, Man and Venereal Diseases." The seriousness of the disease he summed up with the words, "the pox is a pitiless creditor and grants grace to no one." Our own Oliver Wendell Holmes called Ricord the "Voltaire of pelvic literature—a skeptic as to the morality of the race in general, who would have submitted Diana to treatment with his mineral specifics and ordered a course of blue pills for the vestal virgins."

Fournier authored a classic manuscript *Syphilis and Marriage,* and his knowledge of clinical syphilis was almost complete despite the fact that he had no access to laboratory tests. He possessed very good information on the infectiousness of syphilis and did much to encourage other physicians to help prevent marriages between infectious individuals. "The pox like daily bread, is divided between husband and wife," wrote Fournier.

It was in the early part of the twentieth century that the discovery of the causative agent was made by Fritz Schaudinn and Erich Hoffman and the complement fixation was exposed by August von Wasserman. In 1910 Paul Erlich introduced arsphenamine into the chronicles of syphilis' cures.

The syphilization of Europe and the Western world proceeded like a forest fire from 1500 on. Prostitution was a very important factor in its spread, and the disease had a much greater prevalence among the upper classes than it has today. In the nineteenth century, with the advent of the Industrial Revolution, syphilis moved from the leisure classes to the working classes and the cures were the luxuries of the very rich. As living conditions for the average man improved and education was more widespread, he demanded more rigid controls on the infectious spread of syphilis.

Syphilis is a chronic, constitutional, infectious and *contagious* disorder, congenital or acquired, which may attack any tissue or organ of the body. Only the cutaneous manifestations of the disease will be considered in this book, but it must be emphasized that syphilis is a systemic disease and the cutaneous lesions themselves are but a minor reflection of the entire disease. In fact, it was once considered lucky for the individual contracting syphilis to have the skin evidence before the disease had entered the more advanced stages. From the end of World War II until just a very few years ago—during the "penicillin era"—the evidence of the two major venereal diseases, syphilis and gonorrhea, were considered to be of diminishing concern. The wonder drugs—the sulfas and the antibiotics, especially penicillin—were believed to be on the road to eradicating the disease, if caught in time (as clearly as the small pox vaccine had virtually eliminated small pox). But such has not been the case. The rise of venereal diseases, especially among the very young, is incredibly high, and the effectiveness of the wonder drugs has begun to be questioned.

For example, in Los Angeles, the number of syphilis cases rose from 2.9 per 100,000 in 1956 to 17.6 in 1960 and in 1970. The cause of such increases has been attributed to the Pill, which has led to certain increased sexual promiscuity, and also to a carelessness on the part of the young male who does not recognize that the original use of the "Condom" or rubber prophylactic was for prevention of venereal disease rather than birth control. When the girl is "safe" from impregnation, he dismisses his worries and has intercourse without giving due consideration to the possibility that the girl might be the carrier of a venereal disease. The other increase has been among homosexuals. Here the homosexual erroneously believes that venereal disease, like pregnancy, is identified primarily with heterosexual relations, therefore he does not submit to routine examinations. Also, legal and social restrictions make him reluctant to incriminate others and therefore it becomes impossible to isolate and treat those contacted. Regardless of the sources of infection, the two nightmarish diseases which have manifestations in skin eruptions are again in our midst; and in certain metropolitan areas they have reached almost epidemic proportions.

In syphilis, the first evidence of its existence is the initial *chancre* which appears some three weeks to three months after contact. This first incubation period is quite variable in length, as you can see. At least six weeks after the original inoculation, but often considerably longer, the more or less generalized cutaneous manifestations appear, the *secondary* eruption. The manifestations graduate from minor skin phenomena which may simulate several other conditions, to serious or grave illness. The majority of these symptoms are not diagnostic in nature and may consist of such symptoms as sore throat, headache, loss of hair, swollen glands, pains in the bones and joints, and many others.

During the incubation period there is a gradual enlargement of the superficial lymphatic glands. Those nearest the early lesion enlarge first. The enlargement varies from pea-size to nut sized and is hard, painless, indolent, freely moveable with no tendency to break down. Where the primary lesion is on the face (or extragenital) the glands become as large as a small egg.

Acquired syphilis is initiated in a primary sore which may

be evanescent and quickly pass away, especially in women; but syphilis without the warning chancre is very rare. The clinical appearance of the chancre varies with its location, age and accidental features added by infection or irritation. It may originate in a scratch, a superficial abrasion, fissure or herpetic lesion. It may be level with the surface or moderately or markedly elevated. The surface may be scaly, eroded or ulcerated. The common type is the chancrous erosion which begins as a small abrasion that slowly enlarges, becomes oval in contour and is surrounded by a dark red areola. Its surface, at the first is smooth and glossy, later becomes covered with grayish pellicle and exudes serum, which may be tinged with blood. Early diagnosis is most important in the cure of the disease. Beyond the genital areas of men and women, chancres appear most commonly on the lips, fingers, female breasts, tongue, tonsils, eyelids and cheeks. Frequently, the cue is an ulcer which will not heal. In the original stages, it is not usually painful, but sometimes after ulceration sets in, pain ensues—especially when the chancre is in a mucous or tender area.

When syphilis has settled in the human system, the later skin manifestations, which occurs about two years after the original contact, are technically known as *syphilodermata.* Syphilis may be benign or malignant. Usually it is only moderately severe and it is the great imitator of all other skin diseases in its varied manifestations. Usually, however, the lesions are not acutely inflammatory and are slowly progressive. The more general and profuse the eruptions are in the early stages, the more favorable the prognosis. The shades of syphilitic lesions are usually less brilliant than those of other skin diseases, tending to a dull mixture of red, yellow and brown. One of the common color identifications is the color of raw ham highlighted with tones of copper, but one should not attempt a self-diagnosis by any selected color chart. The best aid in recognition is that the lesions are rarely accompanied by itching, burning or painful sensations of any sort.

No portion of the skin is free from the possibility of invasion by syphilis. The disease may from the offset involve the entire skin body or it may rapidly spread from point to point until it finally covers a large area, or it may be limited to one part of the body. For purposes of simplification, the various forms of syphilodermata may be divided into the early types of macular, papular, pustular and follicular eruptions. Macular occurs most prominently about the trunk, shoulders, upper parts of the arms, back and chin. The papular has the same localizing tendency with increased predeliction for the face, palms and soles. The pastular has an affinity for the face and scalp. (Black people are especially susceptible to this type of syphilis). Follicular appears especially on the back and extensor surfaces of the extremities and on the scalp. (It is often mistaken for alopecia areata).

Syphilis is produced by infection, either accidental, intentional, or *in utero.* The germ reaches the blood stream through the medium of the lymphatics and is subsequently distributed through the body. The disease may be, and usually is, acquired directly in sexual intercourse, in kissing, in medical examinations, in nursing at the nipple, or it may be acquired indirectly through the medium of contaminated utensils such as a drinking glass, tattooing needle, hypodermic syringe and other such means. The epidemiclike proportions of the disease today are high among the young people who use drugs and transmit the disease into the blood stream with the use of dirty needles when administering a fix. In the Free Clinics the old dread spirochete, bending and weaving its way like a movable cork screw, is frequently seen under the microscope. It is a delicate organism that requires warmth and moisture for survival; but it is an insidious, evil scourge that has bedevilled man in his sexual pursuits and exploitations.

Syphilis is also congenital, and is transferred to the fetus from the mother rather than the father. Another mode of transmission is the infection of the infant as it passes through the birth canal of the mother who has recently acquired syphilis and has infectious lesions. These conditions, until recently, have been under control—especially among patients who received proper pre-natal care. The syphilitic mother need not produce a syphilitic infant if she is properly cared for and the fetus is protected and treated.

Congenital syphilis differs from the acquired form chiefly in the absence of a primary lesion and greater severity of symptoms. It can cause a premature expulsion of the fetus and there can be active manifestations at birth, but most commonly the manifestations appear within the first four weeks, and no later than three months, after birth. If the child is born with obvious skin lesions, the diagnosis is usually severe and the prognosis—negative, or grave. On the other hand, the child can be born with a good clear skin, be plump and well nourished and the skin manifestations appear at a later date. The breathing of a syphilitic infant is often sufficient to arouse a suspicion as to the nature of the child's disease. The mouth, the vulva and the anus of the syphilitic infant are where the congenital mucous patches usually appear.

The secondary phases of congenital syphilis are evidenced in conditions affecting the cornea of the eye which cause early blindness, the teeth, acoustical defects resulting in deafness, liver and spleen disorders and enlarged bone areas. Neurosyphilis is definitely a part of congenital syphilis and must be recognized as such in the systematic process of the disease, just as if it were acquired syphilis.

The other love goddess disease, *gonorrhea,* named for the infectious germ which carries the disease, is in truth the real "sin" sickness, for it can only be caught through sexual contact. The *gonococcus* is one of the weaker organisms which attack the human body, and it enters through one of the mucous areas—usually the vagina, anus, mouth or eye. The most commonplace area is the female vagina where the bug nestles and grows to maturity sometimes without issuing any symptoms until well imbedded, lustily thriving and infecting all who enter. The early symptoms of burning, itching are often confused with "itching" of the vulva or the anus and unfortunately dismissed as such. Unless there is a visible discharge the infected person believes or likes to believe that the infection is the simple itch—or pruritus. On the other hand, the victim of the latter often suffers agony and humiliation before seeing a doctor in fear that he or she has gonorrhea. I, like many doctors, have seen ghastly cases of vaginal or anal "itch" which has been neglected because of the patient's fear or shame. Gonorrhea in the female can really only be diagnosed by a doctor unless the female knows she has been infected and has reason to suspect the reason for her discomfort. In the male, it is usually quickly recognized. For many years, it was considered a "nothing" disease, an infection one got in the normal routine of a male sex history. Penicillin was the miracle worker, the wonder drug which made gonorrhea a casual, insignificant happenstance. But, today, this is not so. Many people, as we have noted, have an allergy to penicillin. Also, the effectiveness of the antibiotic is weakened by constant usage for minor ailments. Organisms build a resistance to the curing drug. In addition, the type of gonococcus which is now affecting a large number of victims is a rather strong, virulent strain which has a resistance to ordinary dosages of penicillin and other such drugs. Once the infection has set in, it sometimes can never be completely cured—only its worst symptoms are suppressed. It goes undercover, so to speak, and then, when least expected, again rears its ugly head and captures a new victim. The incidences of gonorrhea have so increased—especially among the young—that in the metropolitan areas it could be considered epidemic. Obviously the sexual permissiveness of our contemporary culture, with the use of the contraceptive Pill, the relaxing of abortion laws, and so on, have all tended to make sex not only a necessary function in our day, but a careless custom among many persons. Certainly, if we are going to live a sexually permissive life, we must have an adequate sexual education to know the dangers of the game we are now playing without any set of prescribed rules.

The main purpose of this chapter dealing with the most prominent venereal diseases is to point out the irony in the fact that, despite the fact that your dermatologist is also a syphilologist, most people who become infected with one or another of the various social diseases do not—in the beginning—consult their dermatologist about the cause of their trouble. They are usually seen by a practitioner in one of the other fields of medicine which evolved from the study of syphilis *per se*—and which for many years suffered under the stigma in the eyes of the layman—is often the one doctor to whom the infected person does not turn. Often, the infected person gets to the venereologist by circuitous routes, and frequently after having resorted to remedies suggested by friends and other remedies, many of which can effectively camouflage the actual malady and make diagnosis more difficult. Meanwhile the disease itself is in relentless progression.

I again wish to emphasize that the purpose of these words on skin diseases is to warn you that your skin, being your protector, should not be neglected when it bursts forth and demands your attention. It actually is crying for medical help and you should take heed because many of the diseases as we have shown are nuisances, indications of a more serious internal condition, not contagious but self-infectious, and very often curable, especially if treated properly in time.

In the authoring of a book on skin diseases or in medical panels on the subject, "case histories," as the term is used, are rare because the dermatologist does not have the patient under acute observation for a sufficient length of time to make sincere appraisals. Usually, the skin doctor only sees the patient at times of crisis. Once the emergency has passed, the patient disappears until the skin erupts again.

Certainly there is no legitimate doctor who wishes to increase *hypochondria* in a plagued and troubled world, but on the other hand there is also no doctor who relishes having to treat a serious skin problem which might have been avoided by early proper diagnosis, and less self-administered "home remedies."

Many of man's sicknesses are a combination of physical and mental disturbances. In no area of man's illness is this more evident than in diseases of the skin. The relationship between the patient and the dermatologist commences with the initial introduction, and very often the success or failure of the patient's relationship hinges upon the compatability that is established at first meeting. Most patients are only too willing to unburden themselves as soon as they realize they have a "good listener" in the doctor, and the doctor will not be shocked by anything said, nor will the doctor censure any behaviour which might be at the root of the skin disturbance. You, *the patient,* should be encouraged to talk freely about any matters which concern you, and your doctor should give occasional guidance to further talk with general comments rather than specific questions. A reasonably vague question such as, "Aside from your discomfort physically, how do you feel about your skin condition?" might open up an entire channel of patient-observation which can clue you and the doctor as to the emotional factor involved in the cutaneous disorder which is plaguing you, the patient.

Upon consulting a dermatologist, you should adopt a certain attitude in order to get the most from your doctor by giving him the implements he needs to help you. You should certainly know that no matter what your skin condition is, he has seen and treated much worse and does not see your external blemish as a mark of repulsion, or a symbol of some hidden secret. He sees it for what it is, some form of disease manifested through your most protective organ. You should, then, be prepared to reveal to the doctor of your choice your *early* and *current* attitudes toward:

Yourself: your personality, as well as your body.
Your family.

Your work.

Your social environment, friends, business associates, hobbies, religious affiliations, monetary problems, relations to current world problems such as war, sexual permissiveness, women's liberation, ecology, and so forth.

Your sex life: heterosexual, homosexual (overt or latent), masturbation habits, and anything else that comes to mind.

Past and present physical illnesses.

You and your doctor must then be prepared to handle your skin disease with a realistic approach to such things as:

Conflicts in any of the necessary spheres of adjustment such as change of living environment, or choice of work.

Hereditary factors, or manifestations of your disease in any relatives: how and when the same disease occurred.

Correlation of your skin disorder with periods of stress and strain, traumatic events, time of the appearance of your conflicts and your skin disorder.

All physical symptoms used as defenses against emotional conflicts.

General strength of constitution, physique, all previous illnesses and your own (or parents' or mate's) reaction to such illnesses.

To obtain the best results, your dermatologist should be something of a psychiatrist. He should have a good tolerance for listening and understanding and he must, in addition to knowing the proper medicine to prescribe, *exude confidence.* He must have compassion and understanding and awareness that your skin disease is very often only the external manifestation of an inner depression or anxiety. If he feels the condition is more than superficially neurotic in its origin, he must refer you for further and more extensive mental treatment.

While evidences of skin diseases are quite prevalent in today's neurotic society, evidences of skin diseases among psychotic patients has been endemic. For example, a study of mental patients revealed that the skin in manic patients is usually clear and active, but it may be flushed with the excitement or with anger so easily aroused in these patients. In contrast, the skin of depressive patients not infrequently loses its luster and becomes dry, scaly, and coarse. Hot flashes, burning, tingling and itching sensations are commonplace among depressives. In schizophrenic patients, the skins, generally, are moist and clammy—the result of anxiety.

In 1951, Dr. S. H. Zaidens made a most important contribution to the study of dermatology through an intensive study of skin diseases among psychotic patients. He discovered that the onset of the psychoses was often preceded by the appearance of a skin disorder and that fluctuations in the skin disease were correlated to fluctuations in the psychosis. Very often the confining of the psychotic patient created an improvement in the skin disorder, but as the severe psychosis was improved, the skin disorder reappeared—indicating the patient's return to sensitive reactions. Dr. Zaidens concluded that in actual psychosis the skin is the target of *self-punishment, self-destruction, contamination and infestation.*

In summarizing diseases of the skin we conclude with the facts that few skin diseases are contagious and those that are so only by physical contact through an open lesion in the skin; the look is more abhorrent than the disease; few are fatal if diagnosed and treated in time; most skin diseases are peculiar to certain types of personalities; many skin diseases are pertinent to certain ages of life; a great number of skin diseases are indigenous to climates, personal environment and occupational hazards; some skin ailments are more common amongst one sex that the other, and the color of one's skin is related to the type of skin ailment one is subject to; and, racism does enter into the etiology of skin diseases.

Finally, the all-important thought is that your skin will care for you if you care for your skin!

REHABILITATION IN DERMATOLOGY

The morbidity and disability from dermatological disorders, both acquired and congenital, has an economic value running into hundreds of millions of dollars annually.

Skin is the buffer between man and his environment. When environmental factors irritate his skin, man reacts with inflammation, edema and itching—almost as if to rid himself of the disturbing element. Occupational dermatoses cause the highest percentage of industrial disabilities and *produce the greatest number of man-days of labor lost from non-fatal disease.* Many other cutaneous acquired and congenital defects are also responsible for loss of man-time and man-labor.

In the past four years two centers for the rehabilitation of patients suffering from chronic skin eruptions have been established—one at Louisiana State University and the other at Maryland School of Medicine. The success demonstrated at these two centers has indicated that rehabilitation is an important part of dermatological therapy.

Obviously the primary objective of any rehabilitation program is to assist handicapped or injured individuals in achieving physical, social, emotional and economic independence. The patient's needs must be studied individually in relation to the provision of expert medical care, psychological evaluation, physical restoration and the motivation of the patient.

Rehabilitation seems to involve much more than the 18,500 square centimeters of vulnerability of your skin. As I have attempted to indicate, it involves your essential area of communication with your fellow men; it involves the work you pursue; it involves your sex life—in short, it mirrors your true self. Fortunately, as we know, you are reasonably well protected by the bag in which you live. Actually, rehabilitation embodies those democratic words of idealism that every individual is unique and is entitled to the right to participate in all of the aspects of life and should contribute to society to the fullest of his ability.

A recent report of the Workmen's Compensation Commission shows that 68 percent of the uncontested claims were made by individuals with occupational skin disorders. Forty-eight percent were made by workmen who had occupational dermatoses. Three percent of these people received social security pensions because they were disabled by skin eruptions and 70 percent of these three were under forty-nine years of age!

Figures gathered from LSU and the University of Maryland have shown that many young adults dropped out of school because of severe acne or disfiguring birthmarks.

All of the skin diseases I have listed in this book can be the cause of a deepseated neurosis, or a reason for an individual failing to seek employment or gain it. In addition to its effect on one's earning ability, "bad skin" can be disastrous for the sexual life of the individual, and its damaging effect on psychological make up must not be minimized.

Rehabilitation should begin as soon as proper diagnosis is made and the patient's needs are realized. In the case of a congenital cutaneous, the earlier in life the process is started by the patient's parents, the greater potentials the patient will realize. In occupational dermatitis the procedure should begin as soon as the diagnosis is made and the occupational change arranged.

The length of time for the rehabilitation depends upon the extent of the disease, its response to treatment and the motivation of the patient.

So we begin with an understanding of *rehabilitation* —almost semantically.

Most rehabilitative procedures were developed during World War II. During that time it was clearly demonstrated that most chronically ill persons could be taught to participate in some type of gainful occupation. During the twenty years which have followed, techniques have been greatly refined, and rehabilitation facilities for specialized care have been developed. For the most part these centers concentrated on the care of speech defects, amputees, neurologic disorders, orthopedic disorders and cardiac ailments; but no provision was made for the rehabilitation of patients with chronic skin eruptions. Amazingly, most of these centers would not admit patients with skin lesions, and very few centers had a dermatologist as a consultant. Yet, the person with a chronic skin eruption is potentially a better candidate for rehabilitation than many of those with cerebral palsy, chronic arthritis, or other equally disabling disorders.

It occurs to me that centers should be developed where patients with recurrent skin eruptions can be given comprehensive care, and obviously a trained dermatologist should be an integral part of such a center. Now, two such units have been organized and have had remarkable success in the rehabilitation of the person suffering from an intense skin ailment. Both units were established and subsidized by federal grants.

Such a program requires a study of what we mean by the rehabilition of the individual with a serious skin disorder.* It is your skin and your life, and if, as a dermatologist, I can repair the damage to your skin, what further help can I offer in the rehabilitation of yourself?

The average cost of the rehabilitation of a patient is about $1,000.00 from the time of registration at one of the two established centers to gainful employment. Although rehabilitation on an organized scale has been restricted to the two locations mentioned, there is no reason why rehabilitation cannot be accomplished on a private-patient basis for a private patient. There are complications namely because of the complex nature of the rehabilitation procedures, that the team must function as a hospital which is almost impossible in private practice. The team consists of 1) a dermatologist who surveys the patient to determine all physical

* The cutaneous problems which require rehabilitation include. disfiguring birthmarks, lupus erythematosus, severe acne, psoriasis, nickel dermatitis, cutaneous congenital defects, atopic dermatitis, etc.

defects in addition to the dermatitis; 2) a clinical psychologist who should examine the patient to determine his intelligent quotient, emotional stability, and motivation; 3) a social worker or vocational rehabilitation counselor who determines the patient's vocational potential. This team can determine the rehabilitation of a patient.

An example of rehabilitation is the case of a forty-year-old school teacher with an extensive case of psoriasis. She had been under the care of many competent physicians but did not respond to treatment. In time she became an acute alcoholic and due to her addiction she came to the attention of the law. In time she was removed from her teaching position and became almost indigent, although she came from a family of means and a family dedicated to educational pursuits. They were at a loss for what to do—how to help. Due to her infraction of the law, she came under the observation of her probation officer (a trained social worker), who recommended Alcoholics Anonymous as group therapy for her drinking problem. The woman had an above average intelligence quotient and a genuine love for the teaching profession, but she could not return because of her history. Prior to her arrest for drunkenness, she had an excellent record but under psychological questioning it became apparent that her psoriasis had instigated her drinking problems, which in turn had increased the skin problem. She was persuaded to continue her therapy for alcoholism while arrangements were made for her to be treated with topical medications similar to those previously administered. In time she stopped drinking, gained weight (she had suffered from undernourishment due to excessive drinking and neglecting her diet) and her psoriasis cleared with local medication. In time she returned to her job in the school system, and with the clearing of her skin disorder, stability of her job, and cessation of her drinking problem, she met and married. Today she is living a constructive life.

I cite this as an excellent example of rehabilitation when a common skin disorder brings about a communication problem between one individual and many other nonunderstanding individuals. The results of this kind of problem are more than mere isolation because of the skin disfigurement. They become more psychological than physiological, and as in this case, often result in antisocial behaviour which in turn results in infractions of the law. In this woman's case, disaster revealed a problem which she had been fighting alone. To her friends she merely had "bad skin"—to herself, she had a body of demons which were plaguing her and keeping her from being a useful member of society. With the proper approach and care she was, in truth, rehabilitated. Unfortunately it could have all been prevented with an ounce of care.

REHABILITATION

In evaluating a cutaneous impairment, the physician is playing a role in the ultimate administrative determination of cutaneous disability. Regardless of what type of benefit system is used (government or private) the same type of information should be recorded:

1. Date of onset.
2. Date of recurrence, if recurrent.
3. Date of diagnosis and relationship of patient's disease to existing environment.

4. Diagnosis and clinical condition observed at examination, reasonably correlated with the history given concerning date of onset or recurrence.
5. Supporting laboratory findings, if any.
6. Date of first observation by reporting physician.
7. Date of first inability to perform work.
8. Is the disease a natural disease of life, or is it one which is recognized as environmentally produced?
9. A detailed description of the anatomical changes which have occurred in the patient and a detailed description of the functional changes in the skin in terms of oil glands, sweat glands, acropine glands, hair, pigment appearance, including ability to perceive alterations of heat and cold, touch and pain, and the frequency and severity of pruritis.
10. Limitation of patient to work.
11. Presence or absence of any other physical disorder which might affect skin disorder.
12. Probable response of the disorder to proper treatment. Length of time required for treatment.
13. Standard care required for maximum improvement.
14. Evaluation of the expected duration and the extent of residual impairment.
15. Is vocational rehabilitation feasible, or should patient be advised to seek other means of employment when skin disorder has been rectified?

If your skin presents a problem which affects your ability to work, you owe it to yourself to have such an evaluation made—then abide by the findings. A medical student friend of mine developed an allergy to the metal utensils he would have been obliged to work with had he continued to pursue his career as a surgeon. In medical school he switched when he became aware of his skin problem and is today a very successful practicing psychiatrist. Rehabilitation of skin disorders takes complete communication between patient and doctor. Usually the results are most rewarding.

THE USE OF A MASKING AGENT IN SKIN DISORDERS

In 1936, *Reader's Digest* published an article which told of the granting of a patent to a Miss Lydia O'Leary for the development of a masking agent known as Covermark.

Earlier attempts to patent Covermark had been unsuccessful because, it was contended, the product was merely a cosmetic.

Miss O'Leary personally suffered from a serious birthmark disfigurement—an extensive port-wine stain on the face. Before the judges of the Court of Appeals, Miss O'Leary did a personal application, removal and reapplication of her formula and managed to persuade the Court to grant her a patent in a field where the government had previously denied patents. Miss O'Leary's own story was dramatic and painful. She told of years of unsuccessful efforts to gain employment, emotional rejections and frustrations which were a result of her unsightly skin. She told of the long, tedious study she made until she perfected Covermark. In the decision of the Court, her unsightly birthmark became her legal birthright and brought her fame and fortune. It also gave to the medical world and to the world of blighted human beings a product which is constantly used, and should be used, if your skin is an eyesore and a detriment to you and your pursuit of a happy life.

Unfortunately, Covermark is not generally available at drugstores and other pharmaceutical houses because it is not, in the proper sense, a cosmetic and has to be known by the individual druggist and the patient (usually at the doctor's suggestion).

Also, the application of Covermark for true rehabilitation purposes often requires more instructional time than the usual druggist or salesperson is willing—or qualified—to give. The proper blending of the product with the skin pigmentation of the patient is most essential. At the Louisiana State University Rehabilitation Center, proper applications of Covermark were administered and the results were most successful.

In the past two years ninety-one patients have received individual instructions in the use of Covermark. The majority of the patients had *discoid lupus erythematosus,* vitiligo, scars from various types of trauma, or pigmentary disorders. In many cases dramatic cosmetic results were achieved. One of the most interesting things about the experiment was the readiness with which male patients took to the use of Covermark. Follow-up on the cases showed that men continued the proper usage longer than women. This was probably due to the fact that women are inclined to jump from one cosmetic to another in the hope of finding something more perfect. The findings in the male patients were of satisfaction. One man had spent most of his adult life walking everywhere to get away from the stares and shocked looks of strangers. After learning to apply Covermark, he no longer feared public transportation and has widened his horizons considerably.

Another benefit of Covermark which should be brought to the reader's attention is its use as a sun screen. It is most effective and has not, to my knowledge, been exploited in this usage. It is especially good when there are existing skin eruptions or scars which should not be exposed to the sun. After applying your prescribed medication on the lesion, you can apply Covermark and your skin is protected for the day.

In the use of Covermark, the peculiarly singular psychological attributes of the problems of the skin are revealed. The dermatologist is faced with situations where the attitude and emotional reactions of the patient can have a significant effect upon the results. This area of understanding has been referred to by D. S. Wilkinson in his *Textbook of Dermatology* as the "fourth dimension" of the therapeutic art. Unquestionably, a great part of the successful use of Covermark in the Rehabilitation Clinic is involved with the tender loving care and the human interest on the part of the therapist with the patient. The application, the study of proper color pigmentation, the enthusiasm on the part of the worker, has a great effect on the patient when contrasted with the patient who suffers and applies Covermark alone. Part of the overall problem is the remedying of the skin so that another person will not be turned off but sufficiently turned on to try and discover the real personality of the real person concealed in the bag in which he is living.

CONCLUSION

We are all aware that men and women, since time immemorial, have been interested in improving their appearances. As I have said, cosmetics and cosmetic treatments have been used for centuries to improve the appearance; probably at no time in history has the use of cosmetics been as prevalent, or the range of selection so great, as today. With such wide choice and extensive use, it is to be expected that occasional reactions from cosmetic products will occur.

The vast interest in skin health, skin care, and cosmetics is evidenced by the number of inquiries that come to the attention of the dermatologist.

In addition, it is interesting to note that our nation prefers beauty to bullets. In a recent *Time* article (June 14, 1971), former AAA Administrator E. R. (Pete) Quesada claimed and demonstrated that the common stock of the ten largest companies commonly assumed to be a part of the military-industrial complex was less than that of a single cosmetics firm. The common stock value of companies such as Lockheed, Boeing, and North American Rockwell was found to come to $4,723,814,437, while on the same date the common stock of Avon Products was valued at $5,618,240,682. In 1970 American women spent, with Avon alone, $759 million just to acquire "the look they like."

From reading you are now aware that several features must be considered in the study of the causation of cutaneous diseases, namely: environment, occupation, allergy to food, drugs, animal and plant substances; bacteria, fungi, parasites and viruses; climate and seasons (certain diseases exist only or mainly in tropical countries and other diseases such as psoriasis flourish mainly in winter weather); heredity; race: as we pointed out while very few diseases are prone to attack a certain race it is well known that the preponderance of keloids (excessive scarring)—grows in immense proportion in black people, as does leukoderma. Also, pigmented sarcoma, especially the idiopathic multiple, is often limited to Semitic peoples, but for the most part we know that most skin disorders occur without much selection as to race; age; physological state (especially in women at menstrual periods and during pregnancy and menopause); neuroses; association with other diseases (*xanthoma* with diabetes); internal secretions (disturbances in the sex glands in cases of acne); errors of metabolism; transmission of infectious diseases (most importantly, syphilis).

You now know your skin is one of the vital organs of your body. It is closely associated with the underlying structures and by its situation in covering your body it is brought into intimate relation with the outer world and with other people. It is complex, elastic and sensitive, varying greatly in different conditions of climate, age, sex, health and race and varying also in the characteristics exhibited in different localities upon the same individual. Consequently there is a wide range between the fair skin of the blonde Caucasian and the black skin of the African Negro, between the rosy pink of the infant's palm and the dark brown hue of the genital region of the aged. Your skin varies in pliability and thickness, being delicate and lax over the eyelids, the lips, the prepuce, and much thicker and more firmly attached over the palms and the soles.

With this much knowledge you know that your skin is your individual problem and its care is your personal responsibility. To add to external beauty you like to see, you may experiment for years before you find the most satisfactory external make-up, or you may stumble upon it in your first choice. And, in the cases of skin diseases which are the external eruption of an inner illness, you must work from the inside out, so to speak, whether the problem be organic or neurotic in origin. Your skin cannot be removed from your whole being, your inner self.

To help you with some of the minor problems which affect you and your skin, I have selected a series of questions most often asked by patients and the best simple answer or remedy I can recommend. Perhaps this conclusion will help you to attain the look you like for yourself.

Q: Is there any difference between cold cream and cleansing cream for cleansing the skin?

A: The average cold cream is composed of a cream to help dissolve the fatty skin secretion known as sebum and loosen particles of grime. Other materials facilitate the removal of dirt with a soft towel or tissue. Water drops suspended in the cream give a cooling effect, consequently the name, cold cream. The so-called liquefying cleansers are a variation of the cold cream. They remain on the skin for a short time only.

Q: Please explain the difference between lubricating, conditioning, moisturizing and night creams.

A: These creams are intended to remain on the skin overnight or for a longer period of time than cleansing creams. Their purpose is to promote skin smoothness by relieving dryness and roughness. There are many products on the market. I personally recommend the Nivea creams, and for those indiviudals who do not wish to pay the high prices of expensive cosmetics, good old-fashioned Crisco is very satisfactory. Solid Albilene cream can also be obtained at a much more reasonable price and is the trademark of the actor's profession. It is used both for the removing of heavy theatrical make-up and is applied lightly as a protective cream. To alleviate toughness in a very thick or calloused skin, castor oil is effective, although the odor can be somewhat offensive.

Q: What is the value of rejuvenating creams and hormone creams?

A: Creams advertised as being made of secret products which will make the woman past thirty-five look younger in the face and neck areas are mostly wild promises, conceived in some advertising brain. Royal Jelly from the queen bee is one of the most popular mystical ingredients, followed in popularity by orchid pollen, turtle oil, milk oil, "Formula X-9," placenta extract and milk serum.

If you are bored with your look and have no better way to

spend your money, indulge in any of these products. The results will be the same—nil, unless possibly psychological.

As to hormone creams we know the wrinkling process is of an unknown exact cause. Hormone creams could conceivably act to help counteract the changes that occur between the layers of skin and the supporting tissues. But, there is no scientific data to prove this. It is highly doubtful that one could apply sufficient hormone cream to the body surface to create any noticeable result.

Q: Is it better to use medicated cosmetics than other preparations?

A: The practice of incorporating antibacterial agents into soaps, cosmetics and other toilet preparations has increased steadily through the past years. Hexachlorophene is the agent most commonly used; the names appear on the product package. Their uses are good in the treatment of minor cuts and abrasions, but their use in cosmetics is questionable. In fact, in some instances the brief benefit of safety from bacteria while applied in a cosmetic is far offset by the danger to persons who are allergic to the ingredients.

Q: Is there any type or brand of lipstick which will offset dryness?

A: Most lipsticks contain oil-wax mixtures, lanolin, a staining dye, perfume and other color pigmentations. One study based on the sale of thirty-three million lipsticks indicates that there were 1.57 complaints reported to the manufacturers per million units sold. Each of the ingredients included in the lipstick could create a personal allergy. Your dermatologist can help you solve this riddle, but many women find by simply changing brands they obtain finally the right lipstick with the proper ingredients to avoid dryness and allergies.

Q: Is there any cosmetic line which can be recommended for a sensitive skin?

A: Here, you must consult your dermatologist to discover the cause for skin irritation with the application of cosmetics. There are many manufacturers of cosmetics who have co-operated with the medical profession in the removing of certain agents from their commercial products. These firms supply your doctor with the formulas and by knowing your special allergy he can prescribe the proper cosmetic.

Q: Is it true that certain brown spots on the neck and face can be caused by perfume?

A: Certain perfumes contain photosensitizers which enhance the effect of ultraviolet rays on the skin. Sometimes after sunning at the beach, if one has applied a perfume containing oil of bergamot, such spots will appear. This type of spotty pigmentation is called *berlocque dermatitis.* While it is cosmetically disturbing, it is not dangerous and will disappear in time. Meanwhile the spots can be camouflaged by a masking camouflage such as Covermark or Liquimat.

Q: Is it true that you can get an eye infection from borrowing mascara?

A: It is true. No form of mascara or eye make-up should be borrowed. I personally do not approve of the borrowing of any cosmetic, and most certainly not eye make-up.

Q: What are the different types of hair coloring preparations?

A: Hair coloring preparations are made of 1) analine (organic) products, which include permanent oxidation dyes, semi-permanent coloring preparations and some temporary coloring preparations; 2) metallic salt dyes which are permanent dyes; 3) vegetable dyes which are permanent dyes; 4) acid color rinses which are temporary coloring preparations; and 5) bleaches which remove rather than add color to the hair.

Analine and bleaching products account for most of the sales in hair dye products. All of the organic products are required by law to carry a caution label on the directions and include directions for patch testing. Read this label carefully and you will read: "CAUTION: this product contains ingredients which may cause skin irritation in certain individuals, and a preliminary test should be made first according to accompanying directions. This product may not be used for dying eyelashes or eyebrows—to do so may cause blindness."

Vegetable dyes have probably been in use longer than any other hair dyes. These dyes, which are rarely used today, are: indigo, camomile, logwood and walnut hull extract. The only vegetable dye still used is henna, but it produces only the reddish color hairdressers tend to try to eliminate. Henna consists of ground dried leaves and stems of a shrub found in North Africa and the Near East. The powder is made into a paste with hot water and applied directly to the hair. The chief advantage is safety, as it apparently has no toxic qualities and almost never sensitizes.

Q: How does the consumer tell the differences in different types of hair dye when making the purchase?

A: Carefully check the labeling on the package when making the purchase. All of the organic dyes, both permanent and semi-permanent, carry caution statements and directions for patch testing. The permanent organic dyes require a developer while the semi-permanent preparations do not and include a statement that the results will only last a few shampoos.

You must know that excessive bleaching of the hair, or the radical changing of the hair color which requires intensive bleaching, will in time cause the hair to become harsh and strawlike. Excessive hair damage is not uncommon. This is because peroxide, the bleaching agent, destroys the hair protein as well as the color pigment. However, the damage is limited to the portion of the hair treated and the damage is not permanent; future hair growth is not affected. Obviously if your hair is damaged to this extent with bleaching, the process should be discontinued until new hair is allowed to grow.

Q: Is the teenage practice of straightening the hair by ironing advisable?

A: It certainly is not. The heat can damage the hair temporarily making it fragile and dry and consequently subject to breakage. Also the danger of damage to the scalp by burns is serious and occurs frequently. The three recommended methods for straightening the hair are by 1) pomades; 2) passing a heated comb through the hair (not pressing): and, 3) the use of chemical hair straighteners. In the use of the chemical hair straighteners the most serious damage is to the eyes. At the concentrations used, direct contact between the alkali of the straightener and the eyes can cause immediate, and sometimes premanent damage. This is *not* recommended for home use.

Q: Can the use of hair sprays cause lung damage?

A: There is no proof that there is any relationship between

hair sprays and lung damage, although certain persons (notably hairdressers) develop allergies to certain sprays.

Q: Advertisements suggest that certain treatments will regrow hair on bald heads. Would it be advisable to invest in such products?

A: *Absolutely not!* As I have said, we are all well aware of the fact that bald people grasp at hairs and cherish every fiber. They are ready victims for any promise of hair; they are gullible, easily deceived and often deluded. Recently topical administration of testosterone was recommended as a cure for common baldness. Since this is a highly potent hormone, an indiscriminate use of it could be highly dangerous.

For centuries hair treatments, and remedies claiming to prevent or correct baldness, have been foisted upon the balding public. The most common type of baldness, male pattern baldness, accounts for 95 percent of all baldness. The exact cause is unknown, but heredity, sex, and age are involved in the balding process. Hair-and-scalp "specialists" who show *before* and *after* pictures usually use a person who has suffered from one of the temporary forms of baldness to testify to the power of their product or tonsorial skill. In baldness, diagnosis by a competent dermatologist is required and if there is any satisfactory method of restoring your hair, he will prescribe the treatment for you.

Q: Is it true a person can turn grey overnight?

A: Hair turning grey overnight is one of the great myths of medical folklore and horror tales of the Edgar Allen Poe-vintage. There is no scientific basis for the phenomenon. Hair color results from a deposition of color pigments inside the hair shaft. Unless some material could be formed that penetrated into the hair shaft and bleached or carried away the pigment, there is no basis for the dramatic occurrence. To date no such material has been discovered.

Senile greying of your hair is an irreversible process. If your hair graying results from disease, your color may be restored either temporarily or permanently when you recover from your illness. In these cases the roots of your hair will come in dark and the tips will remain gray or white or you may have a natural frosting of salt and pepper streaks, depending upon the severity of your illness.

Q: Is it true that the "long hair" style, commonplace amongst young men today, is conductive to a continuance of acne?

A: Yes, there is a definite connection and your dermatologist will recommend that if you wear such a hair style you must keep the hair away from your face. Since, as I stated, frequent cleansing is an important feature in the treatment of acne, the young man or woman wearing the current long hair styles might be less inclined to wash the hair with frequency and treat the acne-covered areas since they are covered by the long hair, and consequently prolong a condition of acne.

Q: Are facial isometric exercises helpful for wrinkles and flabbiness and do they improve your face contour?

A: Frankly the answer is a negative one. There are four reasons for the difference between a young face and an old face. 1) The skeletal framework of the face becomes thinner and requires less space with age; 2) the natural lines of expression and action of the face and neck deepen and become more obvious; 3) your skin becomes lax and sags into natural folds and pouches; and 4) the color of your skin changes. These changes cannot be reversed by any form of exercise. The changes primarily involve your skin rather than your muscles and the toning up of the muscles by exercise or massage is of little use and will not benefit the changes that unfortunately accompany aging for any long period of time.

Q: Is it safe to remove age spots with advertised creams?

A: First let me explain that there is no connection between these spots and either age, or liver trouble, although the spots do occur most commonly in older people, usually from overexposure to the sun and wind. They resemble freckles of one's youth except that they are larger, darker and more unevenly spotted and do not disappear in the winter months. No perfect bleach cream exists and the spots should not be experimented with by yourself in a home treatment. You should consult a dermatologist who has several means of removing the spots and he should also be consulted because the dark pigments and enlarged spots might be the first signs of skin cancer produced by years of overexposure to the sun's rays.

Q: Is it harmful to get a suntan if one does not get a sunburn?

A: As stressed right from the beginning of this book, sunlight is the major cause of aging of the skin and skin cancer. Therefore as a dermatologist I must advise anyone against overexposure to the sun. The wave lengths of the solar spectrum that produce new pigment and a suntan are the same ones which cause a sunburn and the effects of wrinkling, laxity, leathery texture and skin pigmentation—all visible signs of aging.

The commercially available "suntan" lotions do not absorb

100 percent of the burn- and pigment-producing wavelengths, but permit a percentage of such energy to reach the skin. Texas Pharmacal Company makes a product called A-Fil Cream, a sun screen, and Sunstick, which are quite satisfactory for use by people with skins sensitive to the rays of the sun. This allows some individuals to stay in the sun and acquire some tan without burning. Your physician can give you some preparations which are stronger and can give you more protection. If you are very light-skinned it is recommended that you consult your doctor before taking on too much sun and destroy in your youth the skin you will have to live with in your old age.

Some individuals get what they call "sun poisoning"—a severe burn in the early summer which prevents them from going into the sun the rest of the summer without suffering extreme discomfort. These individuals have usually developed an allergy to the sun and cannot tolerate any exposure. It is wise to consult your doctor in such a situation. There are internal medications and external creams he can prescribe which might relieve the discomfort so that a reasonable amount of exposure to the sun can be permitted without severe damage and acute pain.

You must remember a sunburn is an actual type of *burn.* It should be treated with wet compresses (ice on the sunburned lips), baby oil and soothing lotions. Little or no clothing should be put on the burned areas and the peeling process should be handled gently to avoid infection.

Patients who suffer from sunning often want to know if a sunlamp is a satisfactory substitute. If it is used properly it is less damaging than the actual sun, but to keep a year-round tan would demand sufficient exposure to make such usage harmful to a person with a light, delicate skin.

And, many patients have asked about the use of the artificial tanning preparations. In general they are safe provided you are not allergic to any of the chemicals used in the preparation. Sensitivity can be recognized by burning or itching following application. Occasionally these preparations, if used constantly, will cause rough and dry skin to develop. Under no circumstances should they be used over a skin afflicted with acne, psoriasis or any of the skin diseases which have open lesions.

Q: Do sleeping pills affect the skin?

A: Sleeping pills are among the list of drugs, including laxatives, headache mixes, antibiotics, tranquilizers and diuretics that can cause drug rashes.

Q: Is drinking bad for the skin?

A: Alcohol may dehydrate the skin for a short time. The effect isn't lasting and won't cause any permanent problems. It can make an itching skin worse since it causes an increased flow of blood to the skin surface. Also in severe cases of heavy drinking, a loss of appetite can occur. At this point poor nutrition could produce symptoms ranging from poor skin tone to cracks in the skin at the sides of the mouth and scaly oil patches around the nose.

Q: Will marijuana have any effect on the skin?

A: At this writing most doctors think not. However it has been suggested that continued use could upset the sympathetic nervous system and stimulate the sebaceous glands. In smoking pot the sense of touch is heightened but there is no skin change. Reports indicate that smoking marijuana decreases your memory capabilities. Concentration is on the present and this probably accounts for the greatly-heightened sensory perception.

Q: Do birth control pills have any reaction on the skin?

A: Many girls have heard their complexions will improve when they begin taking the Pill. This isn't necessarily true. Some girls do notice an improvement in their skin, others complain their skin condition worsened, but cleared up after taking the Pill for several months. Most doctors have noticed a skin change when the girl goes off the Pill. Once the body becomes adjusted to a certain level of estrogen, the backward adjustment can throw your skin off balance. However this is not the most damaging effect of the Pill. In many patients the Pill produces the famous "mask of pregnancy," brown blotches on the forehead and cheeks. The only way to get rid of them is to stop taking the Pill, but most girls would rather cope with the blotches than with an unwanted baby. The blotches can be concealed by the use of sunscreens.

Q: What are the effects of oily foods on skin?

A: A concentrated diet of oily foods is not good for any part of the body—regardless of the skin. Actually there is not a great deal of connection, although doctors do recommend a small amount of oily foods when one suffers from chronic acne. The onslaught of hormones just before menstrual periods and at the age of puberty stimulates the oil glands that with other skin cells blocks pores and forms blackheads. These act as plugs that cause the oil, still coming full force, to collect under the skin. Meanwhile bacteria that are always present on or under the skin go to work on the stagnant oil glands and cause infection. A properly balanced diet is necessary for good health and your skin is the reflection of your state of health. Obviously an oil-heavy diet would produce bad skin.

Q: What causes large pores? What can be done about them?

A: Large pores are usually a matter of heredity. Since oily skin produces large pores, a predisposition to oily skin will often entail this problem. There is not much that can be done. Chemosurgery or dermabrasion can be recommended. Cosmetics can cover to some extent. Astringents, alcohol and ice will help tighten pores temporarily.

So we conclude some of the story of your skin. As you can see, it is a complex story. Skin is a mysterious organ which is only just beginning to be really understood. For the dermatologist and his patient there is a wide unexplored field which has just been entered—the intensive study of skin grafting is an ancient art, practiced as early as 800 B.C. by Hindu physicians. Its modern phase is a search for the answer to your body's rejection of alien grafts. To date no homografts have proved permanent except in some cases of a gamma-globulinemia, among warm-blooded animals of inbred species, *i.e.* certain strains of mice, and between identical twins.

Despite the transience of homografts for practical purposes, they have been used for more than twenty years and their greatest value has been in burn cases in which extensive dermal areas were damaged. Large sheets of split homografts are believed to have saved lives, especially of patients who lose ground daily from debilitation and pain and are unable to withstand a long operative procedure. Homografts may survive over periods of three to ten weeks before absorption;

during this time the patient's condition improves and his own epithelization (covering with new skin) appears to be stimulated so that recovery may occur after the absorption of the grafts. The grafts themselves usually disappear without leaving any noticeable infections, thus leaving the skin clear for planing. It is these advances which have led to the organizations of skin banks in large metropolitan areas, it is through continued research and work that you ralize the importance of your skin to not only yourself, but your fellow man. An oddity in skin grafts was developed by William H. Saunders, M.D., for reducing severe nosebleeds by a small autograft of skin to strengthen the fragile mucous membrane within the nose. In some, the severe nosebleeds stopped, in others the severity was considerably lessened.

So we follow the study of skin with constant interest and surprise, both due to the remarkable variations of character this enormous organ exhibits. It expresses all of our known emotions, weeping with us in our distress and stretching for us in our quest for joyous youth. It suffers and it heals, it tortures and it gives love and sensual joy to the lover and the beloved. It speaks for us in beauty and it mocks us in vulgarity. It is our small universe to discover and to live within in comfort and ease, and even more than the spoken word, it has been since the earliest eons of mankind, our prime polarization of intercommunication.

In a summing up I would like to quote from an eighteenth century panegyric on skin:

> See the Depth of Wisdom of God manifest in the Contrivance of this one Coat; here's Provision for the Body's Safety by Sensation, here's a Brace of Girdle to

Bind up the Whole Body, here's Strainers to separate the superfluous Parts of the Blood, here are Conduits for the carrying off of the strained Matter, here's Provision for Beauty and Ornament, here's a fit Juice to preserve all the Parts moist from drying, here's Prevention of Pain thereby, here's an insensible Veil or Scarf to preserve all the sensible Parts, here's Provision for the Preservation of the Skin of Labouring Men.

Here's to you and your skin.

—Robert Helmer, M.D.